Parkinson's: How to Reduce Symptoms Through Exercise

By Kristine Meldrum, BA, ACE

with Jay Alberts, PhD, and Daniel M. Corcos, PhD

Foreward by International Parkinson's Expert
Bastiaan R. Bloem, MD, PhD, FRCPE

Edited by Cliff Lawson

WHAT PEOPLE ARE SAYING
About Kristine Meldrum's Book

"If you want to take back control from Parkinson's disease (PD), you should stop what you are doing right now and buy this book. The stories at the beginning and end will inspire you with life-changing results for people living with Parkinson's disease. Packed in between these vignettes is everything you need to get you off your butt and find an exercise program that will help you retard the progression of the disease. There are extensive peer-reviewed references, multiple exercise regimens, and recipes for motivation— even the clever idea of naming your exercise program after the name of your favorite drink! Read it from front to back or pick and choose what interests you. No matter how you do it, make these ideas part of your plan for attacking PD."

- Linda K Olson, M.D., award-winning author
person with Parkinson's disease (PWPD),
and triple amputee

"As I read *Parkinson's: How to Reduce Symptoms Through Exercise*, I wish I had had this book available while in active practice caring for people with PD! I would have encouraged them to get the book and find a qualified exercise professional to take advantage of the potential benefits that could be experienced by participating in proper exercise. I encourage others involved in treating or caring for PD or other neurode-generative diseases to read this book and the references noted to understand the possibility of improving their patients' lives and the likely slowing of the progression of their disease.

Not many years ago, scientists believed that the brain stopped changing not long after birth. Now, scientists recognize that the brain can develop new connections, redirect pathways, and even grow new neurons throughout our lifetimes called neuroplasticity. Neuroplasticity and the effect proper exercise has on it are astonishing and well-told in this book. The interspersion of the author's real-life experiences with PWPD and the science and processes involved in attaining the right exercise formula make the book engaging and enticing. It makes you want to hear more of their stories, their outcomes, and how they can accomplish them. The amazing people who persist through the fatigue, sweat, and effort required to reach the levels of exercise needed, coupled with the engaged, knowledgeable, caring exercise professionals, produce neuroplastic changes that become life-changing and apparent to all involved. The results are truly inspiring and a testament to the human spirit."

- R. Michael Collison, MD, AAFP

"This book will serve and support the entire PD community. It has so much great information. I think it covered a broad subject exceptionally well."

- John Ball, PWPD and author of
Living Well, Running Hard:
Lessons Learned from Living with
Parkinson's Disease

WHAT PEOPLE ARE SAYING
About Kristine Meldrum's Book

"This is a must-read book for anyone newly diagnosed or if you've had Parkinson's for years! This book lays out the science behind Parkinson's exercise and explains why it is vital for people with Parkinson's to find an exercise program and stick with it. Exercise is medicine. So pick up this book—and keep your hands up!"

- Kristy Rose Follmar, Co-Founder, Rock Steady Boxing
Three-Time World-Champion Boxcr
2022 Inductee to the Indiana Boxing Hall of Fame

"Denial is a strong facet of our human coping mechanism, particularly when it involves our health. Getting out of denial and into an exercise program as soon as possible is what will do the most good. My biggest message to PWPD or parkinsonism is to let the people around you help get you to the gym—especially on days you want to stay home in bed."

- Dr. Joe Johll, OD, PWPD & Progressive Supranuclear Palsy (PSP)
Exercise kept Joe going for 16 years when most live 6-9 years with PSP

Parkinson's: How to Reduce Symptoms Through Exercise is not only a great resource, but inspirational! I am struck by the incredible dedication and determination of the people with Parkinson's disease and the professionals helping them beat back the disease. I enjoyed the incredible mix of explaining the disease and providing real clinical examples. I thought that was the strength of the book—the back and forth with science and personal examples. I found inspiration in the stories and meaning in the medical explanations. The book is certainly very complete and written with great clarity. The tone and style I thought were welcoming and reassuring—don't wait to get your copy of this amazing book for people with Parkinson's disease.

- Dr. James Collison, MD

"Wow! I found this book compelling. I think that even with my Rock Steady Boxing (RSB) work and my running, my "PD Exercise Cocktail Plan" is missing a few ingredients!"

- Steve Gilbert, PWPD

"What an exceptional job you have done with this book. You will help so many people with the information you have provided. I especially enjoyed the individual journeys of the PWPD you profile in the book. I think that the information will be invaluable."

- Kathy Helmuth, RN and co-founder
of Parkinson's Cycling Coach

COPYRIGHT

DISCLAIMER: All the photographs, figures, and charts have been reproduced in this book with the permission of the relevant photographer/organization or are in the public domain.

CAVEAT AND WARNINGS: This book is intended to help guide people with Parkinson's regarding exercise options to improve their wellness. Before undertaking any course of exercise discussed herein or any variations thereof, a person should consult their own medical professionals and discuss such exercises in detail. If a course of exercise described herein is selected, with the approval of a person's medical professionals, it should be undertaken with the assistance and guidance of those professionals as well as of people trained and certified in exercise procedures (such as trainers, instructors, and physical therapists) who are experienced in working with people with Parkinson's. Adherence to these warnings is a necessary part of this process. Because of the nature of Parkinson's disease and its unique and individualized impact on afflicted individuals, no guarantees, express or implied, are made as to the effectiveness of any treatment described in the book for any individual person.

NOTE: The book's win of the 2024 18th National Independent Excellence Award in the "Fitness" book category and its finalist status in the "Health" book category is a testament to its credibility and the impact of exercise on Parkinson's disease. This recognition reassures the readers, caregivers, and healthcare professionals of the book's quality and the validity of the research and stories shared within.

TABLE OF CONTENTS

DEDICATION

I dedicate this book to my husband, Andy, and my children, Alexa and Zach, for their unending love and support while I wrote this book. Alexa brought me quite a few lattes at 5:30 in the morning and Andy took care of everything else so I could focus solely on writing the book. While I love all my Bernese Mountain dogs, Bruticus never left my side while I was writing.

In memory of Joe Johll

FOREWORD

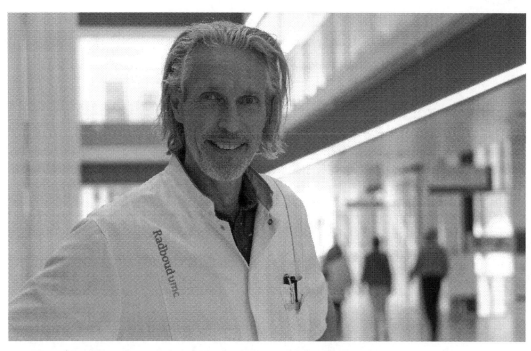

Professor Bastiaan R. Bloem, MD, PhD, FRCPE
Professor of Movement Disorder Neurology
Director, Radboud Centre of Expertise for Parkinson's & Movement Disorders
The Netherlands

Why Every Person with Parkinson's Disease or Parkinsonism Should Read this Book

This new book, *Parkinson's: How to Reduce Symptoms Through Exercise*, is long overdue. Written by recognized experts in the field, this highly readable book comprehensively summarizes the state-of-the-art evidence in the field of exercise and Parkinson's disease.

The book is richly filled with personal stories, both of individuals living with Parkinson's and the scientists who have helped build the evidence to support the merits of exercise as a genuine therapy. Make no mistake, as this book nicely summarizes, there is now a rigorous scientific underpinning to demonstrate that exercise helps to alleviate the symptoms of Parkinson's disease, just as you would expect from a drug that corrects the dopamine deficiency in the brain.

In fact, some of the effects of exercise equal that of a moderately effective antiparkinson drug. The evidence is strongest for the suppression of motor symptoms, such as slowness, stiffness, or tremor, but there is also a steadily increasing body of work that points to improvements in a wide range of so-called non-motor symptoms, including mood and sleep.

And what is even more exciting, there is now emerging evidence to suggest that exercise is not merely helping to alleviate disability, but it may also help to slow the otherwise relentless progression of Parkinson's disease. This contention is now supported by at least two large clinical trials that showed that people with Parkinson's disease who faithfully participate in an aerobic exercise regime at least several times per week suggest that the symptoms of Parkinson's disease in people progressed more slowly than in people that did not involve an aerobic workout. And, additionally, neuroimaging studies in persons with Parkinson's disease have shown that such aerobic workouts are accompanied by beneficial effects in the brain, including the formation of an enhanced functional connectivity between the diseased basal ganglia and the largely healthy cortex of the brain.

> *To my mind, this book is a must read for every person with **Parkinson's disease** who wishes to take more control over the disease by picking up exercise as a new therapy. The book is also a very useful reference for medical professionals who should encourage the people with **Parkinson's disease** seen in their clinics to exercise more.*
>
> **- Professor Bastiaan R. Bloem**

This imaging work is confirming what we had already seen in animals with an experimental form of parkinsonism whose brains were also modified in a beneficial way following exercise. All these findings should really encourage every individual living with Parkinson's disease (or a form of atypical parkinsonism, for that matter) to try to exercise to the best of their abilities.

This wonderful new book summarizes all these different scientific studies and also offers practical recommendations for every person with Parkinson's disease or parkinsonism who now considers starting an exercise regime.

Of course, there are multiple challenges that may interfere with one's ability to exercise, even among those who are deeply motivated. Think about issues such as postural instability and the risk of falls, or factors such as depression or even apathy which may reduce an individual's motivation to participate in exercise. Fatigue is another major challenge for many persons living with Parkinson's disease. This book offers very practical guidance on how to deal with these issues, such as my advice to take some extra medication just prior to a workout so that one can exercise more vigorously, while experiencing less fatigue afterwards.

To my mind, this book is a must read for every person with Parkinson's disease who wishes to take more control over the disease by picking up exercise as a new therapy. The book is also a very useful reference for medical professionals who should encourage the people with Parkinson's disease seen in their clinics to exercise more. As I'm quoted in the book, "We are now in an area where physicians should literally write a prescription for exercise in addition to prescribing more traditional medical interventions such as drugs or surgical interventions."

Read this book if you are interested in learning more about this crucial prescription!

Bastiaan R. Bloem

Bastiaan R. Bloem, MD, PhD, FRCPE
Professor of Movement Disorder Neurology
Director, Radboud Centre of Expertise for Parkinson's & Movement Disorders
The Netherlands

PREFACE

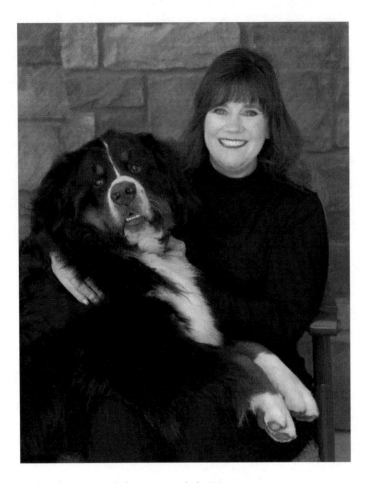

Kristine Meldrum with Tayo

Photo by Laraine Davis

Over the years, I have witnessed the life-changing results that exercise can have for people with Parkinson's disease (PWPD). So, it makes me incredibly sad when I read statistics that say most PWPD don't exercise—even when told to do so by their neurologists, movement specialists, physical therapists, and exercise professionals. I feel worse when I hear that, following a diagnosis, PWPD's activity level drops even lower than people who don't have PD. I feel this way because I know that exercise does help combat PD's deteriorating effects.

I've witnessed that when PWPD start exercising and feel the change for the better, they become ultra-motivated. They want to tackle their disease head-on—which is incredible to watch. The most competitive people I've ever met have PD. It doesn't mean they don't have bad days, but

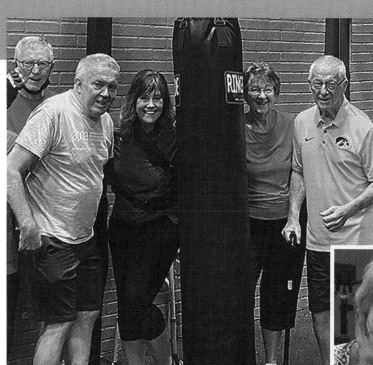

Pictured left to right: Bill Brown, Joe Johll, Kristine Meldrum, Linda O'Hair, and Ed Maahs take a group photo after a Rock Steady Boxing class.

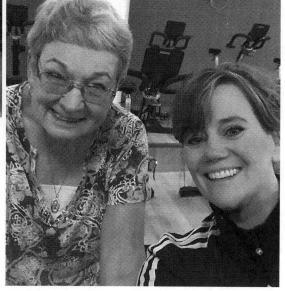

MaryFran Pietig with Kristine Meldrum during a neuro-cycling class. MaryFran loves to cycle and she was surprised how great she feels after a cycling class.

they learn to work through it when times get hard and they keep moving. All of my clients are the most courageous people whom I have had the privilege to guide on their journeys. And they are happy to share their stories with you in this book. Chapters 7 through 10, which are devoted to specific types of exercise for PWPD, conclude with case studies of real people who have used a particular type of exercise in fighting PD.

If you have PD, know someone who has PD, are a care partner, are a medical provider, or want to know what exercise does for the brain, you will want to read this book.

Then perhaps you'll be like my client, Kay, who says laughingly, "Oh, exercise. It's always been the bane of my existence, and now has become my salvation." Kay was immediately surprised and ecstatic

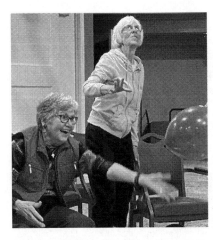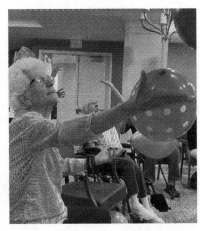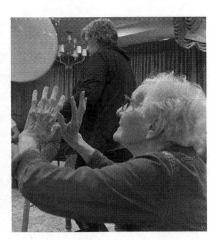

Working with my clients gives me great joy. What I love most is providing an experience they will go home from remembering with a full heart. Exercise should be fun, make you laugh, and want to return. Yes, we work, but it should always be your day's highlight. During a Total HealthWorks demonstration class, participants are multitasking. They say the colors out loud while taping the balloons and reciting the alphabet.

to find out how quickly cycling worked to relieve her symptoms. She felt a huge difference in her motor symptoms immediately after cycling.

"I was surprised by the positive change in how I felt and moved. I feel great working hard, and I know I am helping fight my disease in the process," she remembered. I hope reading the stories in this book will inspire you to undertake the PD exercise journey. When you embark on that journey, you will start to feel great again.

Kristine Meldrum

President, Parkinson's Place Iowa
BA, American Council on Exercise (ACE)
Exercise Professional who works with people with Parkinson's
Iowa Ambassador, Davis Phinney Foundation for Parkinson's
- ACE Certified Group Fitness Instructor
- ACE Senior Fitness Specialist
- Rock Steady Boxing Certified Parkinson's Head Coach
- ACE Approved Parkinson's Cycling Coach
- Certified Mad Dogg SPINNING® Advanced Cycle Instructor
- Certified Mad Dogg SPINPower® Instructor
- SCW Certified Aquatic Instructor
- Total HealthWorks' (THW) Total Parkinson's Instructor
- American Parkinson's Disease Association (APDA) Parkinson's Training for Fitness Professionals

CHAPTER 1

Exercise Is the One Thing That Can Give You Back Control from Parkinson's Disease

"Hopefully, you will, through your own experience, be able to proclaim that exercise really is medicine for Parkinson's disease."

- Jay Alberts, PhD, Neuroscientist, The Cleveland Clinic

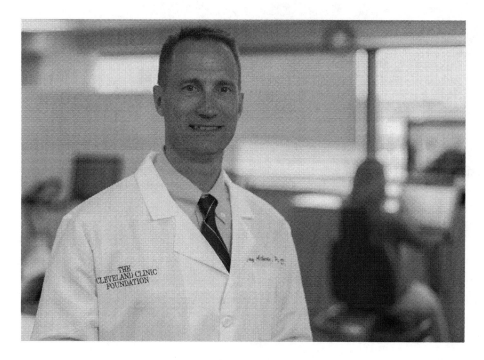

Dr. Jay Alberts, PhD, Neuroscientist

Vice Chair of Innovations in the Neurological Institute, The Cleveland Clinic, holder of the Edward F. and Barbara A. Bell Family Endowed Chair, in the Department of Biomedical Engineering

Research Shows Exercise Improves the Quality of Life for People with PD

"You give me hope" is the phrase I hear most when I explain what exercise can do for a person with PD. After decades of research, high-intensity exercise has been shown to reduce symptoms in people with Parkinson's disease (PWPD). Exercise is also the most promising approach to slow the progression of the disease—particularly if initiated at diagnosis. "Exercise is medicine" is the mantra of the scientist Dr. Jay

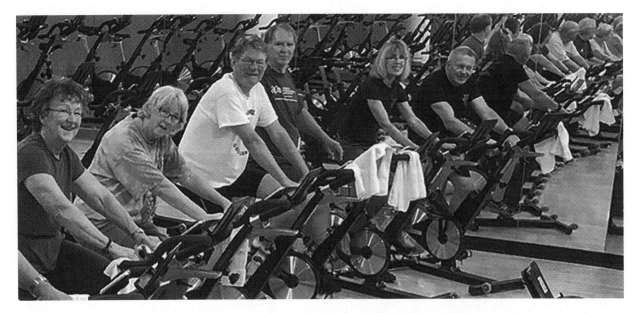

Pictured left to right: Linda O'Hair, Sandy Trent, Jim Clime, Jim Best, Jane Collison, and Joe Johll (many of whose stories you will read about in the book) were all in my very first neuro-cycle class, and they still cycle today.

Alberts, PhD (Neuroscientist, Vice Chair of Innovations in the Neurological Institute of The Cleveland Clinic), who discovered that exercise can empower individuals with PD to take back control of their lives. His quest has been to demonstrate that PWPD can take back control of their bodies from a disease that aims to rob them of their daily functions over time. He says, "The idea is that exercise can potentially spare some of the neurons at risk of dying because of Parkinson's, and thereby slow the progression of the disease."

Implementing Science Into Community-Based PD Wellness Programs

Implementing science-based PD protocols has always been the basis of my neuro-wellness classes. With great success, I followed Dr. Albert's research and methodologies for designing my neuro-cycling classes. His research results for PD show pedaling at a cadence target of 80 revolutions per minute (RPM) reduces PD's motor and non-motor symptoms and may slow the progression of the disease.

While pedaling at 80 RPM may sound fast for a person with a progressive neurological disease, this rate is achievable. I can tell you firsthand it's incredible to watch my clients' resilient spirits and the sheer joy they feel as they get relief from their symptoms after spending a consistent amount of time riding in PD cycling classes.

When my first group of cycling clients were given their initial "Metric Assessments Rides," most pedaled at 50–60 RPM cadences and could only ride for ten minutes of the twenty-minute assessment. Most new clients start here. Six months later, of my roster of twenty clients, the ten people who consistently rode each week could hit the highest speed section of the assessment at 80–90 RPM and had no trouble completing a 45-minute class.

One year later, they all gained leg strength and power output ranging between 100 and 210 watts (they had started between 30 and 50). Best of all, they had better balance, could sleep more soundly, had fewer tremors, had more energy, and felt great that they were taking back control of their bodies.

A Communication Gap Needed to Be Filled

At that point in my career, I decided to publish educational PD exercise articles about the PWPD successes I had witnessed, and I sent those articles to Dr. Alberts. Why not have the articles reviewed by an expert in PD exercise? I will never forget what he wrote to me: "Bringing an effective, laboratory-based, exercise study to community-based programs like the one you are implementing truly represents translational research. Translational research is defined as bringing a treatment or intervention from the 'bench to the bedside.' Unfortunately, the translation often looks more like from the 'bench to the bookshelf' as we publish papers but do not implement the intervention. Your program is translation at its best."

Bringing PD research directly to PWPD and watching it work in the "real world" instead of the lab was essential for Dr. Alberts and me. And it showed that the PD exercise prescription Dr. Alberts was continually researching in the lab was working wonders for PWPD in the community.

Bringing the Scientists' Research to PWPD So They Could Understand Why There Is a Specific Way to Exercise to Reduce PD's Symptoms

With Dr. Alberts' response, I realized I could merge my former profession as a corporate communications and marketing professional with my new role as an exercise professional who works with PWPD. I found my clients wanted to exercise more when they understood what was happening in their brains to produce the results for stabilizing or reducing their PD symptoms. I also received feedback from my clients and other PWPD in the community that there was a considerable gap between what a person with PD hears about exercise and what they actually need to do to relieve their symptoms.

Most PWPD still don't know that exercise can help manage PD symptoms and can potentially delay disease progression, especially if started at the point of diagnosis. Neurologists, family doctors, PD articles, and resources encourage PWPD simply to "be active and exercise." However, when PWPD are "active" and get no results, and their symptoms get worse, they quit exercising, and the disease has free rein to progress faster.

The major reason for this disconnect between general advice and positive results is that few PWPD understand that there is a specific way to work out that will stabilize or reduce PD symptoms. So, I decided to start educating PWPD and others interested in improving PD treatments. Along with publishing articles, I also expanded my certifications to include seven other PD exercise programs in addition to cycling.

Chapter 1

Proactive High-Intensity Exercise Is Medicine for the Treatment of PD

I knew that for my clients' ongoing battle with PD, they needed a complete neuro-wellness program for their continued progress, so I created a single multi-faceted program that includes Neuro-Cycling, Rock Steady Boxing, Total Healthworks' Total Parkinson's, Tai Chi, Neuro-Pilates, and Neuro-Cardio Aqua classes.

For over a decade, I have devoted myself to my PD and neuro clients, and for the past two years, I have been speaking nationally with my presentation *How to Exercise to Reduce Parkinson's Symptoms—the Science Behind Parkinson's Exercise.*

Professor Bloem, Dr. Alberts, Professor Daniel M. Corcos (Professor of Neuroscience at the Feinberg School of Medicine and a professor in the McCormick School of Engineering at Northwestern University at Chicago), and I have a shared vision—one where everyone on an individual's PD care team (neurologists, PD exercise professionals, family doctors, physical therapists, care partners, and of course, the PWPD) agrees that exercise is, in fact, medicine for the treatment of PD, and that exercise needs to be done proactively so that PWPD can reduce their symptoms and feel better.

Exercise Can Profoundly Change the Lives of Those Living with Neurological Diseases

Most of my clients have PD, but I also have clients with other kinds of neurological diseases. And all of them work harder than my clients who don't have a neurological disease. My clients who "work like exercise is their job" are the ones you will be reading about in this book. It takes that kind of determination, dedication, and daily commitment to tackle PD in a way that you begin to slow disease progression and see improvements.

I often remind my clients that "Mr. Parkinson's doesn't take a day off," and they must diligently care for themselves. I have clients who have been living for sixteen years with Progressive Supranuclear Palsy (PSP) when the majority of PSP patients live only six to nine years, and others who walk in the door with a cane and then four months later don't need it anymore.

They are the ones who have kept common side effects from medication at bay (dyskinesia, wearing-off effects, hallucinations, etc.) because they have kept their medication requirements low through exercise. One of my stroke clients is fully paralyzed on one side of her body and yet is able to ride a stationary bicycle at 80 RPM, which has kept her from being in a wheelchair.

And that's not to say that people don't find relief in performing cardio at a lower intensity three times a week, because they do. Lower-intensity exercise helps reduce the risk of disease, improves heart function, improves blood flow, and helps manage high blood pressure—it just doesn't improve PD symptoms.

We also believe medication and surgery are very important. Both of those treatments are vital to helping PWPD be able to exercise. The results gained from PD exercise depend on the individual, the stage of the disease, their consistency in following their exercise program, how they execute the intensity of the training, how well they eat and sleep, and what they want to accomplish. So much more is possible than you ever imagined.

Meet the Scientist Who Discovered PD Exercise: Dr. Jay Alberts

Dr. Alberts, like myself, was inspired by people with PD. As a young undergraduate student, he heard a man with PD say, "I know what I want to do with my hands, but I can't make them do it." That statement transformed Dr. Alberts' thinking as he realized this disease robbed people of control. From that moment on, he wanted his life's work to be helping people with PD regain control. As a result, Dr. Alberts has spent the last twenty years researching PD through deep brain stimulation (DBS), using technology to better understand and treat PD, and understanding how exercise can be integrated into the care model of PD.

Dr. Alberts Has Been on a Twenty-Year Quest to Find the Most Appropriate Exercise Prescription for Individuals with PD

Dr. Alberts has said, "Fundamentally, Parkinson's is a disease that robs people of control slowly over time. To me, exercise is the one thing that gives some level of power back to the patient. I'm a huge fan of deep brain stimulation (DBS) and appropriately provided pharmaceutical medication. They work. But your physicians make all decisions, and they should. How well you respond depends on how good they are, and other factors. Exercise is the one thing that gives the patient control. Exercise is the best thing from a neuroprotective and neurodegenerative perspective for slowing the disease. What better thing can an individual with PD do than exercise to regain control over this disease?"

Ongoing Research to Help Your PD Symptoms

Dr. Alberts speaks globally about PD exercise, deep brain stimulation, and advanced technology for PD. His exercise research evaluated the effects of assisted and voluntary exercise through tandem cycling on PD motor function. These studies found that high-intensity exercise increases activation patterns within the brain. This translates into improved motor function and slowing of disease progression. Dr. Alberts' DBS clinical trials work with PD patients to determine the role of the basal ganglia (brain structures that help control our muscle movements) in movement control. For instance, his research has shown that unilateral DBS provides long-term bilateral motor benefits for PWPD. His virtual reality technology seeks to optimize the method of programming deep-brain stimulation devices.

This Book Is a Roadmap for Getting Results for Your PD Symptoms Through Exercise

The focus of this book is to provide a comprehensive review of the science that supports the concept of using exercise as a complementary treatment approach to PD. As Dr. Alberts and I present these findings to PWPD across the country, we hear the same message, "Why didn't anyone tell us about exercise? I didn't know there was a certain way I needed to exercise to reduce my symptoms."

And while there has been much more information about exercise and PD over the past years, it still hasn't been enough. And there hasn't been a consistent message for PWPD. Scientists, PD organizations, and PWPD want a consistent prescription and vocabulary regarding exercise as a means to help reduce the symptoms of PD.

That is what this book is going to show you. It's a roadmap showing the exercise path to gettting results for your PD symptoms. There is a "formulaic general prescription" for how to exercise to reduce PD symptoms that is based on two decades of research conducted by Dr. Alberts, Professor Bloem, Professor Corcos, and so many other scientists in the PD research field. I have worked with countless clients who have implemented this research and experienced its life-changing results. And we will share testimonials from clients and others who have used these PD protocols to control, stabilize, and manage their PD symptoms.

A Book for Everyone with PD and Their Care Teams

To get the most out of this book, use the information we present regarding PD exercise, in conjunction with the help of a physical therapist (PT) or experienced exercise professional who works with PWPD, to create the best personal PD exercise plan for you. You can read this book chronologically or skip to the chapters that interest you the most, where you can choose from history, science, PD exercise programs, and so forth.

Unlike other books, this one has information for your entire PD Care Team and can be read at any level of detail. *Parkinson's: How to Reduce Symptoms Through Exercise* is a PD exercise education book that teaches people with PD how to manage their symptoms through exercise so they can live happier and healthier lives.

Five Stages of PD

Let's briefly talk about the five stages of PD so that later in the book, when I talk about different exercise programs and at what stage PD they are appropriate for, you will know where to refer back to. In 1967, Hoehn and Yahr (HY) scale was published to define the five stages of PD based on the level of disability. Your neurologist will use this scale to describe how motor symptoms (tremors, bradykinesia, etc.) will progress with the disease. However, PD is as individualized as a disease can be. There is a saying that "Once you've met one person with PD, you've met one person with PD." Each PWPD is unique with the symptoms they experience. Neurologists use the HY scale to measure disease progression. On the scale, stages 1 and 2 are considered early-stage, 3 is mid-stage, and 4 and 5 are advanced-stage PD.

The Stages' Symptoms Defined:

Stage 1: Symptoms (tremor, bradykinesia, rigidity) are mild and generally don't interfere with daily activities. They may affect the person on one side of the body.

Stage 2: Symptoms are more noticeable. Each person is different. They may have tremors, rigidity, and other movement symptoms. They may be affected on both sides of the body and experience walking problems.

Stage 3: Symptoms worsen. Stage 3 is considered mid-stage; loss of balance is the signature of this stage. Turning can lead to falls. Falling can happen more often.

Stage 4: Symptoms are fully developed and cause debilitation. PWPD can walk, but they need a cane or walker for safety. They can no longer live alone and need help with activities of daily living.

Stage 5: Symptoms have rendered PWPD completely debilitated. The legs can become so stiff it is impossible to walk without a wheelchair. Twenty-four-hour care is necessary.

A "gray tusnami" is headed to the USA when 78 Million People Turn 65 and Over in 2030

Currently, nearly a million people have PD in the United States. A "gray tsunami" is headed our way when, in 2030, "all Baby Boomers will be age 65 and over—78 million people" (Gibson "Age 65"). It's projected that by 2040, our country will see an increase in the number of people with neurodegenerative diseases such as it has not previously encountered.

Importantly, PD does not only affect older individuals; many under 50 develop the disease as well. Early onset PD (someone 21–50 years old who receives a diagnosis of PD), which was once considered rare, is also rising. The *Blue Cross Blue Shield Prevalence study* found the following: "While the total number of people affected is relatively small, the prevalence of the condition has grown 53% over the past five years, from 5.5 people per 10,000 commercially insured members in 2013, to 8.4 people per 10,000 commercially insured members in 2017. The likelihood of PD increases with age. While rare, growth of early-onset PD has increased from 1.2 to 2.5 Americans per 10,000" (Blue Cross "Prevalence"). That is an increase of 107%.

A New Study Shows That the Annual Incidence of PD in the U.S. Was 50% Higher Than Previous Estimates

PD is an age-related degenerative brain condition, meaning it causes parts of the brain to deteriorate. It is also a movement disorder. A December 2022 research study titled *Incidence of Parkinson disease in North America* found that the annual incidence of Parkinson's in the United States was 50% higher than previous estimates (Willis 4). The study confirmed that men are twice as likely to have PD, but it also found that women have faster disease progression and a higher mortality rate.

As recently as 2016, prevalence numbers ranged between 40,000 and 60,000 in our country. The study stated, "We established a range of total incident PD diagnoses in North America of approximately 60,000 to 95,000 among adults ages 45 and older. Using the Medicare administrative database alone for this same period suggests an incident rate of PD of nearly 90,000 per annum just for those 65 and older" (Willis et al. 4).

PD Is Now the Fastest-Growing Neurological Disease

More alarming news—PD is now the fastest growing neurological disease. "Neurological disorders are now the leading source of disability globally, and the fastest growing neurological disorder in the world is Parkinson's disease. From 1990 to 2015, the number of people with Parkinson's disease doubled to over six million. Driven principally by aging, this number is projected to double again to over 12 million by 2040" (Dorsey et al. S4).

A study by the Centers for Disease Control and Prevention (CDC) using Wide-ranging Online Data for Epidemiologic Research (WONDER) showed that, from 1999 to 2019, the number of deaths from PD in the United States population more than doubled, from 14,593 to 35,311 (American Academy, Death Rate). The disease has multiple causes, including environmental hazards—air pollution, some chemical solutions used in industrial applications, and particular pesticides. In addition, certain genetic mutations, head trauma, and lack of regular exercise all increase risk" (Rise "Parkinson's Disease").

The countries with the highest use of pesticides and industrialization have the highest rates of PD. "The global use of pesticides is at or near its highest levels. The use of specific pesticides linked to Parkinson disease also persists . . . 32 countries have banned the use of paraquat, which is strongly linked to Parkinson disease" (Dorsey et al. S5).

In his book, *Ending Parkinson's: A Prescription for Action*, Ray Dorsey talks about the hope of ending PD. If we look at the Netherlands for an example of what is possible, then there is indeed hope for the future. The Netherlands has banned many toxins and pesticides linked to PD, including paraquat. And they have watched the number of PWPD go dramatically down. "The Netherlands is one of the few countries in the world where rates of Parkinson's disease are actually waning. A 2016 study found that from 1990 to 2011, the number of cases of the disease 'decreased sharply'" (Dorsey et al. 95).

"A pandemic, as everybody is now painfully aware, is a disease happening worldwide, to which no one is immune. PD fulfills all those criteria," Professor Bastiaan Bloem told *Parkinson's News Today* in a phone interview from the Netherlands. "Parkinson's is now the fastest-growing neurological condition on the planet" (Luxner "Dutch Neurologist").

Professor Bloem Talks about the Link Between Chemicals and PD

"These chemicals were introduced worldwide after World War II, and many are still used today on our fields," Professor Bloem continued. "For this reason, farmers are at a markedly increased risk of developing Parkinson's. If you feed a mouse paraquat . . . it will kill the dopamine-producing cells in the brain. These chemicals are tremendously toxic to the brain and have even been detected in milk, in supermarkets . . . Paraquat isn't the only chemical posing this risk. Trichloroethylene, a solvent used to clean metals and remove stains, has exactly the same effect on human brains. Yet it's still widely used and is detectable in high concentrations in groundwater" (Luxner "Dutch Neurologist").

There are many ways in which people are exposed to pesticides. We automatically think of the food we eat, but many people also use well water, which is often contaminated. In one study, milk was found to contain high concentrations of pesticides (Calahorrano-Moreno 4), and ingesting large quantities of dairy products was linked to the risk of developing PD (American Academy "Pesticide") (Abbott et al. 512). It is not clear yet (research ongoing) (Brown et al. 156–164) (Islam et al. 2–16) to what extent pesticide contamination explains the link between dairy products and PD, and other explanations are also possible.

Whether PWPD should limit or avoid dairy is therefore at this point not certain, and dairy products also have some health benefits, as they contain calcium, which is necessary to maintain bone strength. Many scientists and neurologists suggest that avoiding excessive amounts of dairy products may help to reduce the risk of developing PD (Greger "Dairy Products") (Hughes et al. 49).

Six People in Joyce Gamble's Small Neighborhood Got PD

Joyce Gamble lived in a small community in Illinois. The setting was lovely, filled with families and children. However, adjacent to the neighborhood was a cornfield where crop duster planes regularly flew over and sprayed fungicides and insecticides. During the heavy rain seasons, the water pooled up in the cornfield and then spilled into a ditch that flowed into the first of five ponds scattered throughout the neighborhood. Eventually, this polluted water pooled up around the sidewalks in the area. Kids, of course, love splashing and playing in the puddles. Six people from the neighborhood (including Joyce) were diagnosed with PD. "Oh my God!" exclaimed Joyce. "It carried insecticide right up to our houses. We didn't know it at that time, but science has shown that exposure to certain chemicals can lead to Parkinson's."

Second Opinions Are a Good Idea with PD

People only seem to notice tremors when it comes to PD. There are so many more symptoms, but in Joyce's case, her disease did start with a tremor. She was in her late 60s, having retired from her job as the printing manager for the Department of Economic Development. She described her diagnosis. "I went to this neurologist at one hospital. He told me I didn't have Parkinson's because it was primarily on one side of my body. Knowing what I know now, I'm not sure how he was a practicing neurologist, since PD usually affects only one side of the body. Good thing I didn't listen to him. I went for a second opinion at the Mayo Clinic in Rochester, Minnesota. And sure enough, I had Parkinson's. I mean, seriously. Besides the tremor, I moved like a sloth—unbelievably slow motion. It drove my kids crazy."

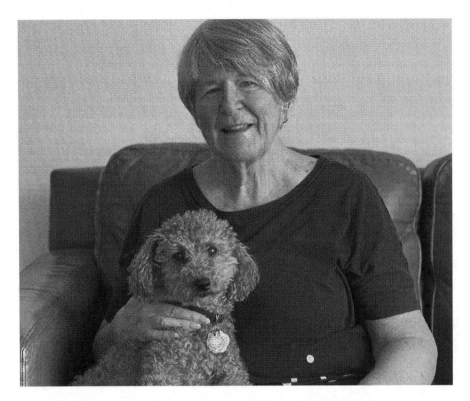

Joyce Gamble says her PD journey so far has been uncomplicated—she attributes that to exercise. She finds great support in her family, friends, and PD community.

Ask about the Makeup of Your Support Group Before You Attend

So, in 2017, Joyce was officially diagnosed with PD and prescribed carbidopa-levodopa. She was told to go home and revisit the Mayo Clinic in three months. Joyce's local neurologist suggested that she find a support group. Joyce had a list and picked one with a familiar name and location. "I have to say, I was in my 60s, but no one prepared me for what I walked in and witnessed. I got there, and the people were so debilitated and in the very late stages of Parkinson's. I was shocked. They rolled a poor man into the room who was laying on a cot because he couldn't walk. I got back in my car after the class and cried for about twenty minutes because it was so bad. So, I didn't see any hope. It was terrible. Finally, I was like, I want to go where people get better. I'm going where PWPD exercise."

Exercise Support Groups Are a Great Choice for PWPD

Ultimately Joyce found herself in a Rock Steady Boxing (RSB) class. "I met Jane Collison (see Jane's story in Chapter 8) at boxing. She is the glue that keeps us all together. Every PD community needs a Jane to keep people informed and exercising—she loves to host 'summer sizzles' and get-togethers." Again, as it had for so many others, boxing brought out the best in Joyce. Attending class three times a week, she felt fantastic. "I think I was in the best shape since I was 35, and that's saying quite a bit for a 60-something-year-old!" said Joyce. "What I liked most about RSB is that there was so much more to it than just boxing. It's so fun, and PWPD and the coaches are there for you."

Joyce's Cocktail with Some Added Infusion of Flavor

When Joyce came to my neuro program, she was ready to try new things. First, we discussed her favorite cocktail—a frozen daiquiri. Her PD Exercise Cocktail Plan™ was named, "My Frozen Daiquiri—No Quackery Mr. PD." At first people scratch their head when they hear "PD Exercise Cocktail Plan™." However, I call it a cocktail because each one is a plan that combines a different balance of exercise ingredients that are best suited to the particular client's abilities and preferences. And, like a person's favorite cocktail, it makes the patient feel better! (see Chapter 5 on PD Exercise Cocktail Plan™s.) Next, Joyce wanted to try cycling, so we added it to her plan along with Total HealthWorks' (THW's) Total Parkinson's class for specific PD work. "Who knew I would love cycling? It was the biggest surprise to me. It's now my favorite thing," Joyce said. She did well right off the bat, especially for someone who wasn't an athlete growing up. Put on Bruno Mars, and she rides like the wind.

Working to Prevent Injuries and Maintain a Balanced Workload

At this point in her life, Joyce must carefully balance her workouts to prevent injuries. She recently has had issues with her knees, and we (the other people on Joyce's PD team) followed up with her physical therapist to ensure that we are working in concert. To address this new development as part of her PD Exercise Cocktail Plan™, we have added progressive strength training two times a week and let her perform rehab cardio with her physical therapist until she could progress back to normal activities. An exercise professional needs to work with physical therapists and keep up to date with the status of clients who are in rehabilitation. I work with a network of physical therapists, occupational therapists, and speech therapists. I send my clients to these other professionals when needed. Likewise, they send me clients—it's a two-way street and a concept that needs to be nurtured.

A PD Journey Requires Lots of Support and Community

Joyce says her PD journey so far has been uncomplicated—she attributes that to exercise. She also thinks it's because of the support she has from family, friends, and her community. "With PD, you just keep going. Now I don't know anybody whose lives have turned out how they thought they would. I mean, everybody has twists and turns down the road of life. But I've learned to go with the flow," said Joyce. However, Joyce does feel that having a group of people facing the same kind of struggle and understanding the complexity of it, including the doctors, makes the most significant difference to her quality of life. "I think having people who know what you are going through is essential. It's too hard to face PD on your own," she said.

Like the Mariah Carey Song Says, "Gonna Make It Happen"

"Exercise is so important at every stage of Parkinson's. I think the first PD support meeting I walked into when I got diagnosed gave me a frightful look at what happens if I quit exercising. So, I don't plan on ever stopping," shared Joyce. "I realize at this stage of my PD, I must work smart. I need to work out enough so that it's helping my PD, but also in a way that I don't injure myself—which is why I like all the different options we have with the PD Exercise Cocktail Plan™. We can make something happen no matter what, because there are so many options."

Always Check with Your Neurologist Regarding Medication Specific to Your Treatment Plan

A comprehensive treatment plan is essential for a person with PD. A good plan will include many things you do yourself, like exercise, eating, sleeping, and drinking enough water. And it might include something that you do with the help of a professional: physical therapy, occupational therapy, and speech therapy or talk therapy. It may also include medications specific to your needs, such as medications that help with movement and others that improve non-movement symptoms such as constipation, urinary dysfunction, or sleep.

Consult Your Doctor for Medications

You and your doctor should work together to determine the optimal medical treatment for your symptoms. Recommendations related to antiparkinsonian medication and surgical approaches to treating PD are beyond the scope of this book. As with recommendations related to exercise, PWPD and their care partners are encouraged to participate actively in the medical treatment of PD. They are encouraged to ask questions of their doctors to fully understand the best medical approach to treating PD.

Exercise Can Help in Ways You May Not Realize

I'm often surprised when I hear PD clients say they didn't know there were side effects to medication if the dosage got too high or if they are on the medications too long—side effects like dyskinesia (uncontrollable movements of the face, arms, legs, or torso), confusion, nausea, hallucinations, or compulsive behaviors. And yet, one of the most amazing things about exercise for PD is that, when it is done in concert with a neurologist, it can help keep medications at lower dosages for longer periods of time.

Study Shows Exercise Keeps You Out of the Hospital

A 2022 report titled *Effect of Exercise and Rehabilitation Therapy on Risk of Hospitalization in Parkinson's Disease* (Kannarkat et al. 2022) shows that exercise dramatically changes when PWPD end up in the hospital. The report said, "Exercise may reduce hospitalizations in PD through reduction in overall frailty, reducing falls, and improvement of medical comorbidities. Increased exercise duration and intensity correlate with reduced odds of hospital encounter" (Kannarkat et al. 498-99).

How Do We Prepare for the Coming Changes?

We read and hear amazing PD exercise benefits from many sources. Yet I often wonder, "Why aren't the PD exercise classes overflowing with students? Where's the demand for more exercise professionals who work with PWPD to help guide the nearly one million people with Parkinson's disease in the United States? How do we prepare for the massive onslaught of future diagnoses?"

Don't Wait until Your Symptoms Get Bad to Start Exercising

If I had a dollar for every PWPD who said, "I wish I could go back in time and start exercising the day I got diagnosed. I could have pushed off the progression of my disease. Why didn't I listen when my doctor said exercise?" Or "Why did I waste two years in denial? I should have been exercising to fight against this disease." I would have a lot of dollars.

Many people still don't even know they could have been exercising to control their PD. Or that there is a certain way they need to exercise to help slow disease progression or reduce symptoms. And they only found out about exercise after the fact when the symptoms appeared or got worse.

You miss out on a window of opportunity to potentially put a pin in the disease's progression if you don't start exercising as soon as you are diagnosed. And the harsh truth is that this disease accelerates quickly with inactivity toward an earlier death—the international PD expert will explain this in Chapter 3. The good news is that it's never too late to start exercising. And you can get results no matter what stage of the disease you are in—if you start exercising.

Please Take Note as You Read This Book

You will read many case studies in this book about people who achieved incredible results through exercising. Their results may be different from your results. These stories are meant to inspire you and show what some of my clients and others have accomplished using various forms of exercise. Your results may vary. Listen to your doctors, physical therapists, and exercise professionals. Before engaging in any exercise program, discuss the program thoroughly with your doctors, and always get consent when required by a new exercise program.

Never Give Up without a Fight When You Have PD

Courage, faith, and a deep love of family kept Joe Johll fighting a long, monstrous battle. Joe's story began when he, a Midwest optometrist, decided to move his practice from a southeastern town in Iowa closer to the capital city of Des Moines. At the time, he was experiencing extreme fatigue and other symptoms. He and his wife, Gail, thought these symptoms were from seven children and the stresses of moving both a practice and a home.

Those Dreaded Three Words . . . It's Parkinson's Disease

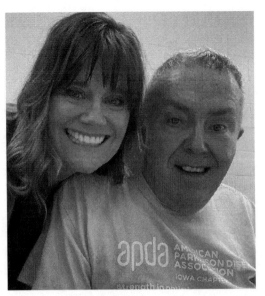

Kristine Meldrum and Joe Johll.

However, as time passed, a gut feeling told them to get him further checked out. They met with a Des Moines neurologist who diagnosed Joe with PD. Of course, this news was devastating for Joe and the family. They were amid multiple significant life changes. Having to face a life-altering illness that gets progressively worse over time was daunting. But if there is one phrase to describe Joe, it is that he is the "ultimate fighter." He was not going down without one heck of a fight.

"I was unhappy about the diagnosis since there is no cure for PD, and no medications worked for me. But I was determined to fight. Once I found out exercise was the one that could combat this disease, exercise became my mission," Joe stated.

His Exercise Of Choice—Rock Steady Boxing

Joe quickly found his exercise of choice: Rock Steady Boxing, a non-contact, boxing-based fitness curriculum for PWPD. He loved everything about it—the camaraderie, the workout, and especially how it made his symptoms feel better afterward. So even though he had a hectic work life and family schedule, he made sure he went to his boxing classes three times a week. But six years into Joe's diagnosis, his symptoms were not getting better. They were getting worse. And they were not following the typical progression of PD.

A Trip to the Mayo Clinic Brought New Information

Joe and Gail went to the Mayo Clinic in Rochester, Minnesota, for a second opinion. After filling out tons of paperwork and getting MRIs and PET scans, Joe had one crazier test—which turned out to be not so crazy.

Joe said, "I remember it was a topical color dye painted all over me. It would confirm if I was positive for Progressive Supranuclear Palsy (PSP) if it turned a certain color. And it did, indeed, turn red—which was the PSP color. I felt relief because we finally had an answer. But utter despair because it's a horrible disease. My wife knew I would be researching my new diagnosis like I was authoring a thesis paper."

Joe Thought PD Was Bad . . . Until He Heard It Was PSP

The progression of PSP is much faster than PD. Whereas PD can be a slow progression over the course of twenty or more years, PSP is like PD on steroids. Most people with PSP are in a dependent-care facility within three to four years of diagnosis. And heartbreakingly, they die within six to nine years.

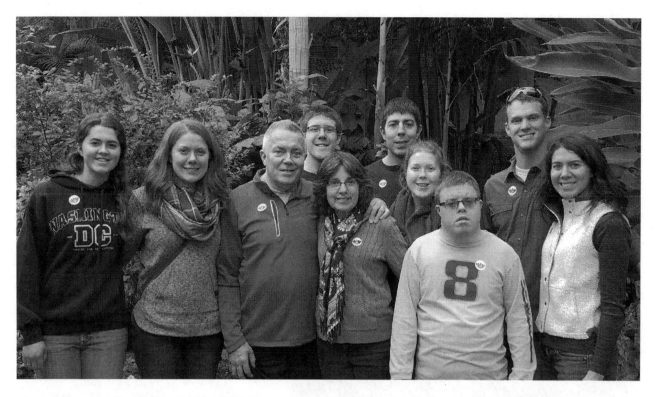

Pictured here are Joe Johll and his wife, Gail, and family at The Botanical Center in Des Moines, Iowa.

At this point, Joe was already at year six of his PD diagnosis (which going forward would be a PSP diagnosis) and focused all his efforts on beating the odds—exercise became his full-time job. The neurologists at the Mayo Clinic had told Joe that exercise was the only thing that could help him, particularly since medication did nothing for him. And remember Joe's wife saying he would write a thesis upon diagnosis? Well, Joe researched everything he could about PD exercise, since it was the only option for him, and he then put it into practice.

Joe Trained Like an Athlete to Beat Back His Disease

Joe was fortunate to have many wonderful coaches during his journey. When I became Joe's exercise coach, we created what we playfully called his Margarita Fight Back PD Exercise Cocktail Plan™ (see Chapter 5), which consisted of Rock Steady Boxing two days a week. He wanted to increase his cardio level to include two extra days of aerobic-endurance exercise, so he chose neuro-cycling. Joe knew he could sustain four days of aerobic endurance workouts, a crucial component for helping to push off his disease progression. In addition, Joe had always loved to do progressive strength training. We decided to have him work with a personal trainer to incorporate strength training two days a week to combat rigidity, balance, and cognitive skills. Joe loved to lift heavy weights. On his strength days, he also added a THW Total Parkinson's class several hours after he finished strength. At the end of the week, Joe took one day off.

Chapter 1

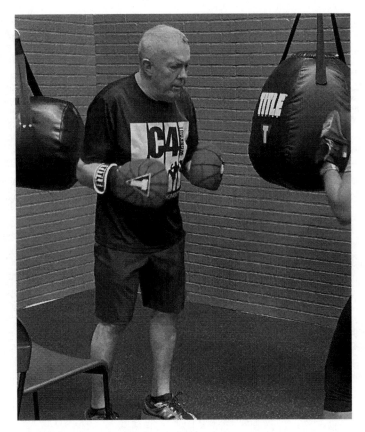

Joe's love for Rock Steady Boxing never changed over time. He couldn't wait to box and see all of his friends.

PWPD Are Individuals and Need to Be Coached as Such

As Joe's exercise coach, I can honestly say I have never met anyone who worked out as hard and consistently as Joe. He trained like an athlete. But he always listened to his body when it told him he needed to pull back and rest. When I tell Joe's story, I sometimes get pushback and the proverbial, "That's too much for people with Parkinson's," or "That's overtraining," from a few coaches. It is not—it truly depends on the individual. And then, I tell them, "Joe pushed off his disease—one that typically takes people's lives within six to nine years—FOR SIXTEEN YEARS!" And their jaws drop.

Joe said, "I am living proof that working out as aggressively as a person's health will allow, prolongs your life. I'm still here punching bags at year sixteen. That is because, one, I work hard at exercise; two, I have absolute faith in God; and, three, my love for my family drives me daily."

It Took a Pandemic, PSP, and Pneumonia to Knock Him Down

We ran into a snag when the 2020 COVID-19 pandemic stopped the world in its tracks. I should mention that during eight of the preceding years, Joe also had bouts of pneumonia twice a year. And that is a significant complication—many people do not survive PSP or PD when they get pneumonia. Joe recovered each time and got back to the gym. However, in November 2020, he contracted pneumonia and ended up in the hospital. Unfortunately, while hospitalized, he also got COVID-19. The combination of PSP, pneumonia, and COVID-19 took its toll on Joe, and he was sent home to hospice in December.

My Main Thought Was, "This Man Needs to Move, Now."

Hospice care is compassionate comfort care (as opposed to curative care) for people facing a terminal illness with a prognosis of living six months or less. Care is based on their physician's estimate if the disease runs its course as expected.

However, I knew Joe had other ideas. He wasn't one to give up without a fight no matter what life threw at him. A few of us from class visited Joe, and everyone discussed what to do. I could tell by the look in his eye that I was right. He still had a fire burning in them. My main thought was, "If this man doesn't move, we're going to lose him."

And I said out loud, "Joe needs to move. Can we get a physical therapist here?" Gail explained that since Joe was on hospice, no one could come in and Joe couldn't go out. I saw Joe's expression from the corner of my eye, which was one of complete despair.

The Look in His Eyes Said He Wasn't Ready to Throw in the Towel

The look in his eyes confirmed Joe wasn't ready to die. He still wanted to live. While driving home, I decided to work with Joe if no one else could. By the time I got home, I had received a text from Joe.

He wrote, "Help, I'm trapped in my body, and I can't do this by myself."

I texted him back, "Don't worry, Joe, we're going to get you out of this."

And we did.

First, I started moving Joe's body, and then we began walking and stretching. Later, I added chair boxing. And when he was ready, I added resistance training to his workouts. Sandy Trent, my stroke client, would come to Joe's house with me, sometimes sitting in a chair and boxing with Joe. He loved it. Joe just laughed with us.

Month by month, we kept working steadily. And on October 1st (ten months after he was released into hospice care), he graduated from hospice and went straight to the gym. Joe was so happy. He couldn't wait to return and see all his friends. He had missed everyone so much.

Chapter 1

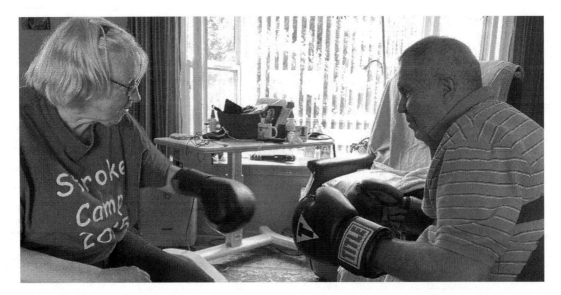

On some days during Joe johll's time in hospice, Sandy Trent would come with me to Joe's house and work out with him. Pictured here, they are seeing who can shadowbox the combos faster during a fun warm-up.

Complications Came Back to Joe's Journey

Dysphagia (having trouble swallowing and speaking) can be a common part of PD and PSP. Joe had struggled for years with both speaking and swallowing. While at the hospital during COVID-19, he had a nasogastric (NG) tube to help with nutrition, and then before leaving the hospital, he had a percutaneous endoscopic gastrostomy (PEG) procedure—a feeding tube placed through his stomach. Joe was still eating and drinking when he came home from the hospital, and of all his favorite things, Joe loved to eat. However, swallowing became an even worse issue. And after Christmas that year, he could no longer physically eat.

It Was Worth Every Minute, Knowing He Was Fighting to Be with His Family

Some people can do well just eating through a feeding tube and improving their quality of life, but Joe wasn't one of them. He didn't do well with a feeding tube at all. In fact, he took a turn for the worse. It broke our hearts to say goodbye to Joe in April of 2022.

Some people ask, "Was it worth it for him to work his way out of hospice?" To which I reply, "Absolutely, YES!" Joe was 64 years old. He was a dear husband, father, parishioner, and friend. He had another year with his family—another Thanksgiving, Christmas, birthdays with all seven children, and another wedding anniversary with his wife. He saw his first grandchild, Joseph, born and named after him. Joe worked his way out of hospice, which enabled him to see his first grandchild and spend time with him and the rest of his family. His grandson was named Joseph, after Joe. In the picture, Joe holds Joseph while Gail watches—life's most precious moments.

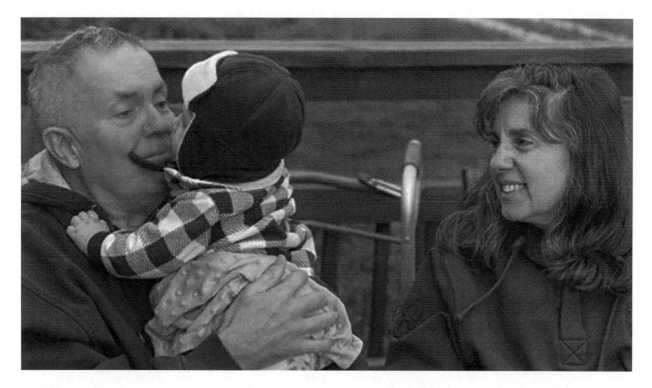

Joe Johll worked his way out of hospice, which enabled him to see his first grandchild and spend time with him and the rest of his family. His grandson was named Joseph, after Joe. In the picture, Joe holds Joseph while Gail watches—life's most precious moments.

The Power of Exercise Demonstrated by a Courageous Man

Joe Johll was an inspiration to everyone who knew him. And it's not just because he could leg press over 300 pounds on his strength days. Or that his biceps looked like Popeye's when he did his bicep curls. He showed his love for his family throughout his life and passed that love on to his PD friends.

Joe Never Gave Up, He Refused to Back Down

Friends and family were Joe's biggest motivators and why he fought to ensure that they were cared for even when he struggled with a rare and downright mean disease. He refused to back down, no matter what PSP threw at him. Joe was a walking testimony to what the power of exercise can do for people with PD or parkinsonism. When he kept falling, Joe got up. When he had to go to a walker, Joe still went to the gym. When he had to go to a wheelchair, Joe was wheeled into the exercise studio. When he ended up in hospice, Joe said, "When can I do some wall pushups?" Everyone who knew Joe loved him and was inspired by him. He showed us to keep going no matter what PD or PSP had to say.

Chapter 1

CHAPTER 2

The History of Exercise in the Treatment of PD Symptoms

"I have no choice about whether or not I have Parkinson's.
I have nothing but choices about how I react to it.
In those choices, there's the freedom to do a lot of things
in areas that I wouldn't have otherwise found myself in."

- Michael J. Fox

People Noticed Her Tremor and Didn't Bother to Tell Her

During Carol Harvey's parents' anniversary party in 1994, her sister noticed that Carol's hands had a tremor when she was taking her parents' photograph. Carol, who would later become my client, was just 33 years old. However, the sister didn't bother to tell Carol about this observation, and Carol didn't notice it herself. Instead, she went on with life, and nothing out of the ordinary happened, that is, until a church choir event two years later in 1996. Carol was on stage holding a microphone with her right hand, and her right hand was swinging uncontrollably back and forth to the point that she had to grab it with her left hand to make the swinging stop.

"Denial is More Than Just a River in Egypt"

Since PD ran on her mom's side of the family, Carol worried about the disease being genetic—though there is only a 10-15% chance of getting PD through family genes (Education Fact). She bought a 23AndMe Genetic Test Kit, which returned a result saying she did not have a PD gene. However, she still made an appointment with a neurologist the following week. The verdict from the doctor came back saying she had an "essential tremor," a nervous system disorder that causes rhythmic shaking that is not related to PD. Carol was relieved. PD was not something she wanted to hear, at 35, as her life sentence. However, deep down, she felt the tremor was PD. She used to say, "Denial is more than just a river in Egypt."

Carol Was Young When She Was Diagnosed, and PD Exercise Was Still in the Dark Ages

Time only increased the "essential tremor" symptoms, and, before Carol knew it, the PD discussion was back on the table. That "unwanted visitor" was planning to stick around this time. Carol was overwhelmed, and rightly so. She had four young boys close in age, one of whom needed care twenty-four hours a day. She had stopped working as a nurse to stay home and care for him. Carol had a lot of balls in the air and was trying to outrun her PD. Carol was symptomatic with PD in 1996 and diagnosed in 1997—unfortunately, still the Dark Ages of PD exercise (1899-2009) (Alberts and Rosenfeldt S22). Over the next several years, her symptoms got worse.

Something had to give, and it would be Carol's fear of deep brain stimulation (DBS) surgery. At the time, her fear was justified; DBS was still a relatively new type of brain surgery that was not approved for PD until 1997. Still, when her doctors recommended DBS surgery to help her symptoms, Carol decided to go ahead with the procedure in January of 2006.

Her husband, Roger, who is an internist with a specialty in infectious diseases, refused to leave her bedside after her surgery. He wasn't going to let anything happen to her, even if it meant going toe-to-toe with the head nurse (which he did) and obtaining authorization from the hospital administrator to stay with his wife. Thankfully, the surgery went well, and Carol recovered from her DBS surgery. Carol had a successful DBS procedure, and it helped with her dystonia (a movement disorder that involves involuntary muscle contractions) and tremor.

Her Sister Called and Told Her to Get to a Rock Steady Boxing Class ASAP

Twenty-six years later, Carol still feels that DBS was the right call. The surgery got her symptoms under control so that she was able to function. When her sister called in 2017, and said, "Pick yourself up a pair of boxing gloves, and find the nearest Rock Steady Boxing (RSB) affiliate," Carol did just that. "I just remember they put me in this safety harness that attached to the ceiling and said, 'Okay, jump!' To which I replied, 'This momma DON'T JUMP!'"

There is something to remember about exercise as a therapy for PD. One of the earliest studies titled, *The Forced, Not Voluntary, Exercise Improves Motor Function in Parkinson's Disease Patients* found that the good results one feels only last for about four weeks after you stop exercise, and then the disease takes over, and the PWPD quickly starts to lose ground (Ridgel et al. "Forced" 2009). Carol had felt this phenomenon at various stages in her life when she couldn't exercise. During this period, Carol began falling, and her balance was so bad that she didn't even want to jump with a safety harness. However, after months of training at RSB, Carol not only jumped off the ground but also performed jumping jacks, high knees, jumping rope, and so on.

When Carol started to train with me, she wanted to continue with RSB, but we added neuro-cycling to her aerobic workouts and a THW's Total Parkinson's class for mind and body work. To this day, there is little that Carol can't do. On National Squat Day, she did 450 squats. Her new phrase became, "This momma not only jumps, but she jumps high!" Carol found that once she started to work out, she felt great both physically and emotionally, her symptoms were manageable, and she found her people—other PWPDs with whom Carol could share the daily ups and downs of managing their disease. She had a group to go out with, have parties, and exercise daily.

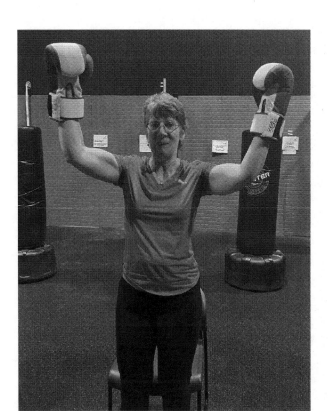

Carol Harvey has been battling PD for 26 years. She has done it through perseverance, a good sense of humor, and daily exercise.

Watch Out, She's Bionic With a Twist

Carol's drink of choice was gin and tonic. Her PD Exercise Cocktail Plan™ became Carol's "Gin and Tonic . . . I'm Bionic . . . With a Twist" (see Exercise Cocktail Plans, Chapter 5). That describes Carol completely. She loves challenges and trying new things. Carol was a competitive athlete growing up. So, I was not surprised that Carol would love progressive strength training. She worked with a personal trainer for several years and made exceptional gains in strength, balance, flexibility, and mental fortitude.

Carol will be the first to tell you that she has lived through twenty-six years with PD by kicking its butt daily with exercise. She's truly unstoppable. She managed to raise four young boys, one of whom needed twenty-four-hour care, while waging a continuous battle with PD. Her enduring spirit inspires everyone. And she never gives up, regardless of what challenges life hands her. She also gives to everyone around her—she has a special way of making sure people are taken care of in a quiet and thoughtful way.

They Thought Sitting Was the Best Thing for People With PD . . . Boy, Were They Wrong

PD has long been recognized as a distinct human ailment. In ancient India, Ayurvedic medicine referred to PD as "Kampavata"—"kampa" meaning "tremor" in Sanskrit (Mandal "Parkinson's History"). The earliest reference to bradykinesia [slowed and impaired movement of the limbs] dates to 600 BC. Evidences prove that as early as 300 BC, Charaka [one of the principal contributors to Ayurveda] "proposed a coherent picture of parkinsonism by describing tremor, rigidity, bradykinesia, and gait disturbances as its components" (Ovallath and Deepa 566).

The Greek physician Galen described what was almost certainly PD in the second century AD. It was the English physician James Parkinson whose name was given to the disease by William Sanders in 1865. In 1817, Parkinson had described cases of the disease in a paper titled *An Essay on the Shaking Palsy* (Parkinson 1817). He is credited for accurately describing the disease as an "involuntary tremulous motion, with lessened muscular power, in parts not in action and even when supported; with a propensity to bend the trunk forward, and to pass from a walking to a running pace: the senses and intellects being uninjured" (Parkinson 223). See a historical timeline of PD exercise in Figure 1.

PD EXERCISE HISTORY TIMELINE
How We Got Here

Dr. Jean-Martin Charcot

600 BC
Ayurvedic medicine referred to PD as "Kampavata"—"kampa" meaning "tremor" in Sanskrit."

300 BC
Charaka described the components of parkinsonism as tremor, rigidity, bradykinesia, and gait disturbances.

Dr. Sir William Richard Gowers

1850
FIRST RECOGNITION THAT MOVEMENT AIDS IN SYMPTOMS FOR PARKINSON'S DISEASE (PD)
Frenchman Jean-Martin Charcot used movement as a treatment for PD. "His shaking chair" gave relief to PWPD.

1899
THE DARK AGES OF EXERCISE AND PD
Sir William Richard Gowers published his *Manual of Diseases of the Nervous System* in 1899. It marked the beginning of the Dark Ages of PD exercise–because Gowers sent everyone home to sit.

1975
Parkinson's Medication
Carbidopa/levodopa became commercially available.

1980s
LOW-INTENSITY EXERCISE
In the 1980s, to recommend that PD patients perform low-intensity chair exercises, although there was little evidence for their efficacy.

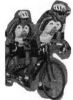

A young neuroscientist, Jay Alberts, cycled tandem with a PWPD, Kathy Frazier, on what turned out to be the 2003 PD exercise discovery ride.

Early 2000s
PD Animal Research
Positive results from animal studies ushered in the age for use of exercise as an additional treatment with medicine for PWPD.

2003
PD EXERCISE DISCOVERY RIDE
A bike ride across the state of Iowa "(RAGBRAI)" led to PD cycle clinical trials at The Cleveland Clinic.

2007-2009
PD CYCLE TRIALS BRING FORTH LANDMARK STUDY FOR PD EXERCISE
Research centered on how the brain controls movements proved that high-intensity cycling improves PD motor movements and function.

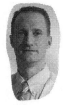

Dr. Jay Alberts

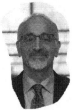

Professor Daniel M. Corcos

2012-2015
SPARX2
High-Intensity Treadmill Exercise on Motor Symptoms in Patients with De Novo Parkinson's trial showed that people who exercised at high-intensity delayed the progression of PD symptoms; moderate-intensity workouts had no effect.

2018
PARKINSON'S BECOMES THE FASTEST GROWING NEUROLOGICAL DISEASE

2015-2019
PARK-N-SHAPE STUDY, NETHERLANDS
Aerobic exercise at home through "Exergaming" system showed PWPD will follow through on their own.

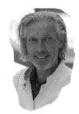

Professor Bastiaan R. Bloem

2023-2028
SPARX3
The $20-million SPARX3 study has 29 sites in North America and one site in Canada with 370 participants. The study the study aims to provide more concrete evidence that high-Intensity exercise slows the progression of the signs of PD.

2016-2018
PARK-N-SHAPE PHASE II STUDY
Fifty-six of the original Park-N-Shape participants study went on to participate in the *Aerobic Exercise Alters Brain Function and Structure in Parkinson's Disease: A Randomized Controlled Trial*. Results showed that high-intensity exercise stimulates neuroplasticity in the brain, slows brain shrinkage, and makes new connections to the healthy part of the brain.

Figure 1. PD Exercise Timeline

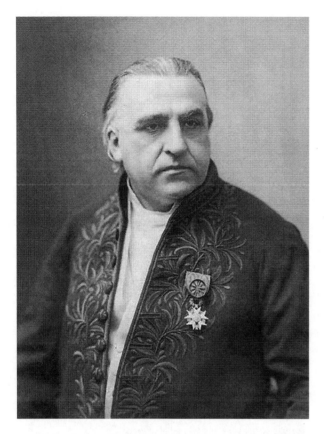

Father of Neurology, Frenchman Jean-Martin Charcot
(*Public domain from the Bibliotheque-Naionale-de-France*)

First Concept of Using Movement for PD Treatment Practiced by the Father of Neurology

The man who first observed that some type of movement, be it active or passive, could potentially diminish a motor symptom was Frenchman Jean-Martin Charcot (1825-1893). Charcot practiced at the Salpětrière Hospital in Paris and is considered the "Father of Neurology" (Kumar et al. 46). Largely because of him, neurology became its own field. Charcot expanded on James Parkinson's "definition" of PD and distinguished PD from other diseases that also had tremors—including multiple sclerosis (Goetz 28). "Charcot and his students described the clinical spectrum of this disease, noting two prototypes, the tremorous and the rigid/akinetic form" (Goetz 29). In fact, he was the first to classify parkinsonism-plus syndromes. Charcot popularized the term "Parkinson's disease," rejecting the earlier designation of paralysis agitans (a less common term for Parkinson's disease) or shaking palsy, because he recognized that Parkinson's disease patients are not markedly weak and do not necessarily have tremors (Goetz 27).

Chapter 2

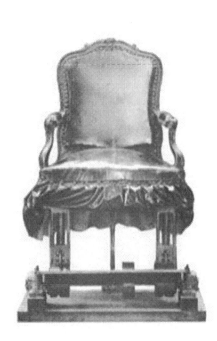
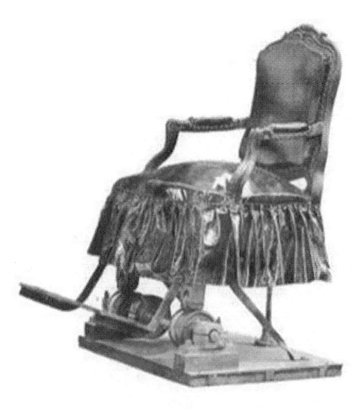

Charcot's "shaking chair." This automated vibrating chair was considered somewhat a success. Patients were prescribed daily thirty-minute sessions and, after five or six sessions, reported that they felt better.
Public domain from the Bibliotheque-Naionale-de-France

Charcot Noticed That PWPD Were Better after Train Rides, Long Carriage Rides, or Riding Horses—Each a Form of Movement of the Body

Charcot turned his concept of movement into a treatment for PD after he observed that his patients were remarkably better after a long carriage, train, or horseback ride. Around 1890, he came up with a vibratory therapy for the management of PD that was essentially an electric-powered "shaking chair" (*fauteuil trépidant*) (Charcot 1892).

He immediately had his patients try the chair and took observational notes. "As soon as he comes down from the trépidant-chair, the patient feels lighter; his stiffness is gone; he walks with more ease than before" (Charcot 823). Charcot goes on to write, "An almost constant phenomenon—the nights become good; the patient, who before was agitated incessantly in his bed, sleeps a quiet sleep, which brings him great satisfaction" (Charcot 824).

According to a peer reviewed paper titled *The Universal Prescription for Parkinson's Disease: Exercise,* "Goetz [Christopher G. Goetz, Professor of Neurological Sciences and Pharmacology at Rush University Medical Center] and colleagues developed a similar vibratory chair and were unable to replicate the initial observations of Charcot in a randomized trial . . . it appears the initial observation [Charcot] may have been placebo. Nevertheless, Charcot's suggestion that movement, albeit passive, may be useful in treating PD could have started a revolution in the use of exercise to treat PD" (Alberts and Rosenfeldt S22).

Into the Exercise Dark Ages for PD Patients

Unfortunately for many PD patients, another neurologist in England, Sir William Richard Gowers, followed similar treatment strategies and came to a much different conclusion. Unlike Charcot, Gowers "stressed the negative effects of mental strain and physical exhaustion, advocating that life should be quiet and regular, freed, as far as may be, from care and work" (Gowers vol. 2. 607). His approach was more medicinal. He prescribed the following: "For tremor, he used hyoscyamine and also noted arsenic, morphia, conium (hemlock), and 'Indian hemp' (cannabis) as effective agents for temporary tremor abatement" (Gowers vol. 2. 607). This sent the field of PD exercise treatment down a long and dismal path. Once Gowers published his *Manual of Diseases of the Nervous System in 1899* (Gowers vol. 1. 1886), neurology entered the Dark Ages of PD exercise because Gowers sent patients home to sit, an action that accelerates disease progression.

Imagine the progress that might have been made if neurologists had followed Charcot's suggestion that movement was the right path for treating PD and, beginning in the 1860s, had started exploring movement and exercise to help slow the progression of PD. But that did not happen, and it would be more than a century before aerobic exercise for PD treatment was given serious examination.

More Than a Century After Charcot's "Shaking Chair" Experiments, PD Exercise Is Rediscovered at a Bike Ride

The 2003 RAGBRAI (Register's Annual Great Bicycle Ride Across Iowa)—a cycling event in which thousands of participants bike across Iowa—forever changed treatment philosophies for PD. A young research scientist, Jay Alberts, organized a group of PWPD cyclists and their care partners and convinced them to join him in the trek across the state. Many were riding on tandem bikes. One couple had made it only one day into the seven-day ride and they were already heatedly debating the optimal approach to making it across Iowa on their tandem bike. Dr. Alberts suggested to the wife, Cathy, that she finish the ride on Dr. Alberts' tandem to preserve her marriage. They rode along, pedaling at a furious pace, and Cathy proclaimed at the end of each day, "I don't feel like I have Parkinson's."

Even more surprising to Dr. Alberts was that her handwriting improved as the ride continued—Cathy, like many PWPD, experienced micrographia—small and illegible handwriting. At a stop along the way, she wrote a birthday card to one of her teammates. The script was larger and more legible than usual, which prompted Dr. Alberts to ask, "Who wrote this birthday card?" Cathy proudly responded, "I did! Isn't it amazing?"

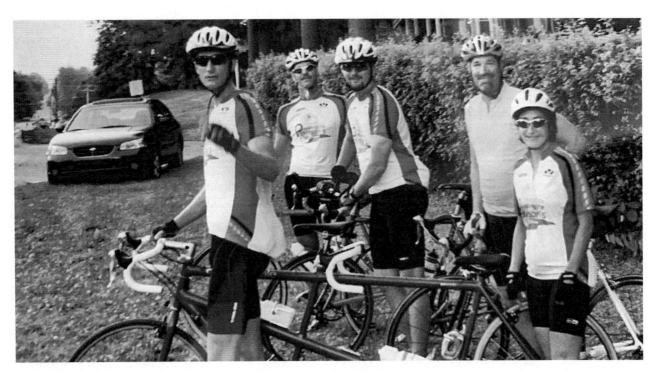

The infamous ride across Iowa that led to helping so many PWPD. Pictured left to right is Jay Alberts, Ralph Frazier, Joel Alberts, Gary McCarthy, and Cathy Frazier.

Was It Homemade Pie in Iowa or the Cycling That Made PWPD Better?

Initially, Dr. Alberts chalked this improved handwriting up to the pie and ice cream RAGBRAI is famous for delivering at each town stop—the desserts make people wonder if Iowa is heaven. However, Dr. Alberts continued to ride tandem bikes in PWPD-organized rides in other less heavenly states, and the responses from the PWPD were consistent: "I don't feel like I have PD when I am on the bike," was a typical comment. Likewise, with so many other PWPD symptoms improving on subsequent rides, Dr. Alberts realized he needed to move beyond the therapeutic potential of homemade gooseberry pie and investigate the effects of high-intensity exercise on PD symptoms.

From the Cornfields in Iowa to Clinical Trials at the Cleveland Clinic, PD Exercise Emerges From the Dark Ages

That research journey progressed from the Iowa cornfields to clinical trials in 2007. The purpose was to determine how the brain changes during exercise to improve motor function in PWPD. The *Forced, Not Voluntary, Exercise Improves Motor Function in Parkinson's Disease Patients* study (Ridgel et al. 2009) compared two cycling groups: one group riding tandem bikes at a "forced-effort (FE) pace" (pedaling at a higher intensity than they usually would by themselves) and a second group riding at a "voluntary-effort (VE) pace" (pedaling at their own pace). Both groups improved aerobically. However, the Unified Parkin-

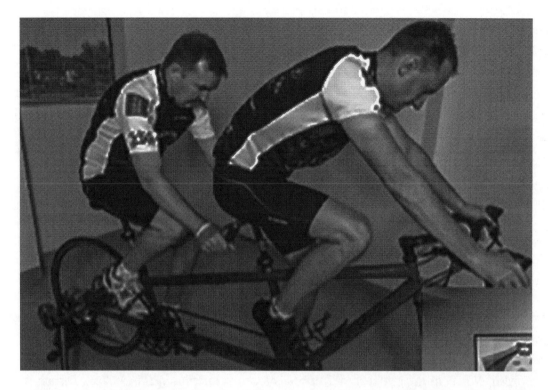

In 2007, a man with PD, left, and Dr. Jay Alberts in the first CYCLE Clinical Trial testing to see if Dr. Alberts' theory based on the RAGBRAI would prove true (whether PD motor symptoms would improve through high-intensity cycling on a tandem bike in the laboratory setting).

son's Disease Rating Scale (UPDRS) motor scores for the FE group improved by 35%, whereas patients in the VE group did not exhibit any PD motor symptom improvement (Ridgel et al. 600).

The FE group also substantially improved their overall motor function—balance, tremor, stiffness, and bradykinesia (Ridgel et al. 602).

Only the Forced-Exercise (FE) Group Improved PD Symptoms

There are three important aspects of the cycling trial to understand. First, at the point in time in medical science that the clinical trials were undertaken, the notion of having PD patients complete high-intensity exercise was an outside-the-box approach. Hence, the fact that the VE group had relatively low pedaling rates was not surprising because they had never been encouraged to move quickly. Second, both groups exhibited improvements in cardiovascular fitness, so PD patients can derive other health benefits from high-intensity exercise in addition to improving PD symptoms. Finally, an important aspect of gaining benefits from exercise may be related to the target cadence in addition to getting your heart rate into a specific aerobic zone.

If Your Goal Is to Keep PD Symptoms Under Control, There are Specific Things That Have to Happen When You Exercise

Three scientific studies in this book (Ridgel et al. 600-608) (Schenkman et al. 219-226) (Van der Kolk et al. 998-1008) indicate that PWPD need to be working at a higher intensity (MHR) to help with PD symptoms and potentially slow disease progression. I know that "high intensity" sounds difficult or even impossible, but I will explain shortly why it's achievable, individualized, and not as hard as you think it will be to get to the target 80% of maximum heart rate (MHR) level.

Those living with PD often become discouraged from regular exercise because they are not experiencing results. Then they quit exercising because they don't think it's working. They hear random advice rgarding intense exercise from various sources: "It's okay just to walk." "Just do what you can." "Yes, you can leisurely ride your bike." That just isn't the case if your goal is to manage your PD symptoms or slow disease progression. You must break a sweat or feel breathless to know you are at 80% MHR.

Dr. Alberts' Landmark Study Started a Chain Reaction for How PD Patients Are Treated

The 2009 study, *Forced, Not Voluntary, Exercise Improves Motor Function in Parkinson's Disease* became a landmark study (Ridgel et al. 600-08). It was one of the first proclamations that exercise should be part of the prescription for PWPD. This paper also sparked scientific studies (Rigel et al. Dynamic 1-8) (Alberts et al. 177-86) (Segura 1-11) on exercise for PD. Dr. Alberts' breakthrough research helped reverse the common practice of prescribing rest for PWPD, and it would dramatically change how PD patients would be treated.

It Was Just the Beginning of the Search for the PD Exercise Prescription

After completing the 2009 study, Dr. Alberts started a series of PD cycling trials, ranging from *Variability in Cadence During Forced Cycling Predicts Motor Improvement in Individuals with Parkinson's Disease* to *It Is Not About the Bike; It Is About the Pedaling,* and more—all part of the search for additional evidence that high-intensity exercise improved motor symptoms and slowed disease progression.

Cycling Worked Better Than Medicine in Research Study

Dr. Alberts then investigated more precisely how exercise works in the brain like medicine. At the time, scientists didn't fully understand the mechanisms of exercise or medication used for PD. The most exciting finding was that the forced-exercise (which today we call high-intensity-exercise) group "improved patient's motor functions clinical ratings by 51% compared to 33% in patients who received medication" (Beall et al. 195). *The Effect of Forced-Exercise Therapy for Parkinson's Disease on Motor Cortex Functional* PD *Connectivity* study compared the effects of FE and medication using both resting and continu-

suomotor task fcMRI (functional connectivity MRI). Ten patients with mild to moderate PD completed three fMRI (functional MRI) and fcMRI scanning sessions randomized under the following conditions: on PD medication, off PD medication, and FE + off medication. Blinded clinical ratings of motor function (a Unified Parkinson's Disease Rating Motor Scale-III exam) indicated that FE and medication resulted in 51% and 33% improvement in clinical ratings, respectively" (Beall et al. 195). The findings went on to say, "Exercise has a strong effect on baseline cerebral blood flow, with increases in the motor cortex of up to 20% up to 30 min after exercise" (Smith et al. 2012 cited Beall et al. 2013).

> *FE (Forced exercise) improved patients motor function clinical ratings by 51% compared to 33% in patients who received medication.*
>
> *- "The 2013 **Effect of Forced-Exercise Therapy for Parkinson's Disease on Motor Cortex Functional PD Connectivity** study"*

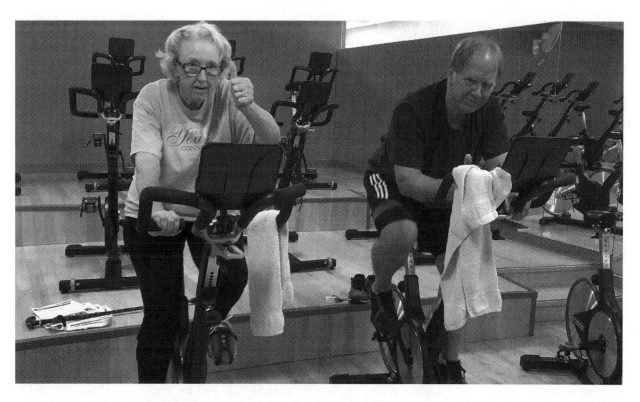

Sandy Trent, left, is my stroke client who is paralyzed in one half of her body, rides with Jim Best, right, my PD client. It took Sandy quite some time to be able to ride at higher cadences, but she is able to ride at 80 RPM even with her condition. Sandy gets four hours of mental clarity after a neuro-cycling class.

Chapter 2

After Living Forty Years in A Brain Fog, Sandy Finds Four Hours of Mental Clarity After Each Cycling Class

The cerebral blood flow study explains why my stroke client, Sandy, gets four hours of mental clarity after a cycling class. Sandy is completely paralyzed on one side of her body. It took us a few tries to get her up onto the bike, but once there, she increased both speed and time. Initially, she rode at about 50 RPM. However, after six months of riding five days a week, Sandy could pedal consistently between 80-85 RPM and easily ride for 45 minutes.

She explained, "Since having a massive stroke at twenty-six, I was paralyzed on both sides. I worked for years to relearn how to use my left side when it became functional after being paralyzed, which is not my dominant side. I thought it would be impossible to ride with my paralyzed leg. However, with the help of God and Kristine, I experienced a true miracle. And within six months, I could hit 80 RPM and my watts got up to 80.

"I had the strength to stand up in the saddle after two years of cycling—which was my personal goal. Nearly forty years later, after living in complete brain fog, I experienced mental clarity for the first time after my first cycle ride. I started cycling five times a week for those four precious hours when I could function like a normal person."

Science Study Finds Cycling and Medicine Use Similar Pathways to Produce Symptomatic Relief

The Motor Cortex, Functional Connectivity study referenced above found that although cycling and medication are very different ways to treat PD, they work in the brain similarly to relieve symptoms. "Medication and FE are two very different therapies that can improve symptoms in PD. The therapies also led to similar alterations in the pattern of functional connectivity. These results suggest that these therapies, despite being very different in application, likely use similar pathways to produce symptomatic relief. There was no statistically significant difference in the change from baseline UPDRS between FE and medication" (Beall et al. 197).

At This Time, No Drugs or Surgical Approaches Can Slow Disease Progression for PD

Despite advances in modern medicine and surgical approaches for PD treatment, therapies to help slow or stop disease progression have remained out of reach. "Neurodegenerative diseases are characterized by progressive damage to the nervous system, including the selective loss of vulnerable populations of neurons, leading to motor symptoms and cognitive decline. Despite millions of people being affected worldwide, there are still no drugs that block the neurodegenerative process to stop or slow disease progresion" (Schmidt et al. 571).

Early animal studies indicated that high-intensity, but not low-intensity, exercise had neuroprotective properties (Zigmond et al. S42) (Tajiri et al. 200). When studies showed it was helpful to PWPD, it prompted short-term human exercise studies; (Herman 1154-8) (Fisher et al. 221-9), and then, several large studies that examined the long-term effects of aerobic exercise on motor and non-motor symptoms in PWPD. A study titled *Phase I/II Randomized Trial of Aerobic Exercise in Parkinson's Disease in a Community Setting* found improvements in aerobic fitness, motor symptoms, and quality of life after following a six-month walking program in PWPD (Uc et al. 413). However, *The Study in Parkinson Disease of Exercise Phase 2* (SPARX2) (Schenkman 219-226) examined the safety, feasibility, and potential efficacy of long term high-intensity aerobic exercise in slowing PD progression in PWPD.

"If you have Parkinson's disease and you want to delay the progression of your symptoms, you should exercise three times a week with your heart rate between 80 to 85 percent maximum. It is that simple," said then co-lead author (SPARX2) Professor Daniel M. Corcos, PhD, in an interview with Marla Paul of *Northwestern Now*. (Paul "Intensity").

A Treadmill Study by Wendy Kohrt Was the Model for SPARX2

Just as the great bicycle ride across Iowa inspired research for PD cycle exercise, an earlier treadmill study looking at age and heart rate in older adults was the foundation for PD treadmill exercise. A study titled *Effects of Gender, Age, and Fitness Level on the Response of VO2 Max to Training in 60-71-Year-Olds* (Kohrt et al. 204-11) showed two significant findings:

1. With this type of vigorous exercise training, 80-85% MHR on a treadmill, people aged 60 to 71 years-old adapts to endurance exercise training to the same relative extent as in young people, and this adaptation is independent of gender, age, and initial level of fitness (Kohrt 209).
2. "When subjects were divided into three groups by age (60-62 yr, n=42; 63-66 yr, n=43; and 67-71 yr, n=25), there were no differences among the groups in the relative increase in Vo2max . . . The rate of increase in Vo2max was not dependent on age" (Kohrt et al. 207).

The SPARX2 team took this study, re-designed it for PWPD, and ultimately made a monumental impact on PD exercise.

Groundbreaking SPARX2 Trial Demonstrated That High-Intensity Endurance Exercise May Be Key to Slowing Disease

SPARX2 was a treadmill study that included 128 PWPD aged 40 to 80 years (Schenkman et al. 219-226). They were divided into three groups (Usual Care, High Intensity, and Moderate Intensity) and exercised four times weekly for six months. One group exercised at a high intensity (80% to 85% of maximum heart rate), another group exercised at moderate intensity (60% to 65% of maximum heart rate), and the Usual Care group was not given any instructions with respect to exercise. The exercise groups were compared with the Usual Care group who were instructed to do what they normally do (Schenkman et al. 220).

Chapter 2

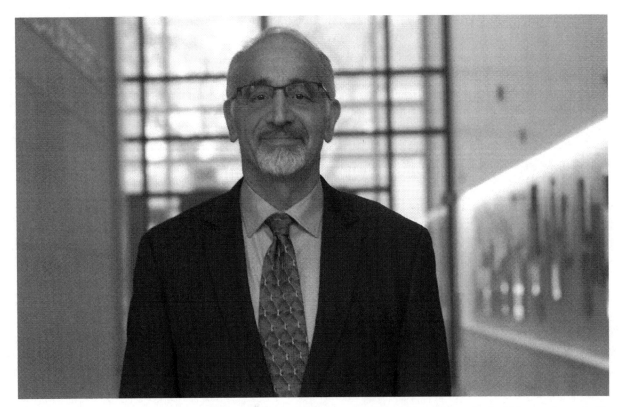

Professor Daniel M. Corcos, PhD, professor of Neuroscience at Northwestern University in Chicago, is currently the lead investigator for the SPARX3 study (see Chapter 7) and was the co-lead Investigator for the SPARX2 study).

Groups Exercising at Other Than High-Intensity Did Not Reduce PD Symptoms

"The study results suggest that people who exercised at high intensity delayed the progression of PD symptoms, while moderate-intensity workouts had no effect," said Dr. Deborah Hall, then associate professor in the Rush Department of Neurology and an author of the study. The important point to understand is that the moderate group and the usual care group did not slow down their PD symptoms.

SPARX2 Is One of the Most Pivotal Research Studies for PD Exercise

The SPARX2 report has had 35,809 views, 221 citations, and a score of 631 on Altmetric—a science company that tracks where published research is mentioned online (news outlets, blogs, tweets, Facebook, Wikipedia, Google, and so forth.) The data provided by the SPARX2 study was so impactful that it provided the stimulus to write a Phase 3 Clinical Trial (SPARX 3), which is supported by the National Institute of Neurological Disorders and Stroke (NINDS). Over the next few years, the SPARX2 study will become a citation classic and has already ensured its place in PD exercise history.

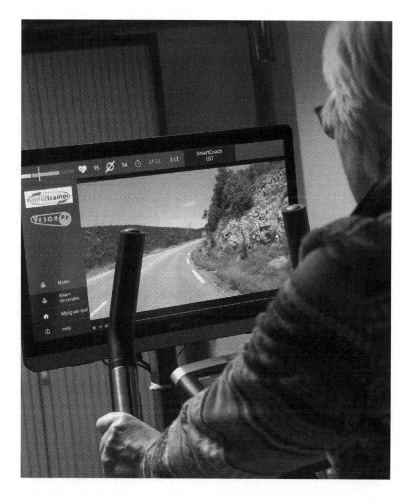

"Park-in-Shape" participant follows the program design at her home in the Netherlands. It was one of the early clinical trials that was taken out of the hospital setting and into the patient's home.

Park-in-Shape Clinical Trials in the Netherlands Move Out of Hospital Environments and Into Patients' Homes

The Effectiveness of Home-Based and Remotely Supervised Aerobic Exercise in Parkinson's Disease: A Double-Blind, Randomized Controlled Trial (Van de Kolk et al. 2019) from the Netherlands was one of the biggest game-changers for PD exercise. It was exciting because it took the trial out of the hospital setting and into the PWPDs' homes. One goal was to see if people would be motivated to work independent of a clinical setting, and they were monitored and had contact with trial personnel over six months.

The researchers divided 130 PD patients into two control groups, and they were part of the study from 2015 through 2017. The aerobic-exercise group had stationary bikes with gaming equipment ("exergaming")—a form of motivation. The non-aerobic group performed stretching, flexibility, and relaxation exercises. This group also received a motivational app. Both groups worked out three times a week for 30-40 minutes, and

Chapter 2

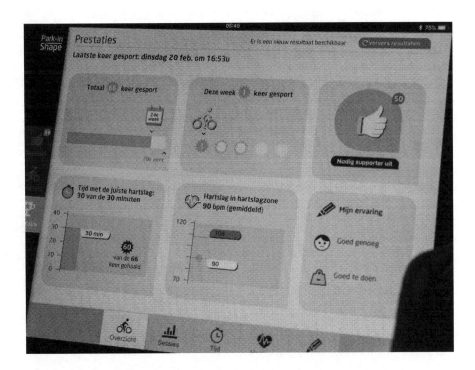

The aerobic-exercise group had stationary bikes equipped with gaming equipment called "Exergaming" as a form of motivation. In addition, important information such as heart rate, time at work, and progress for the week was tracked in real time.

they worked out on their off periods of medication. The trial looked at motor and non-motor symptoms, quality of life, physical fitness, and adherence to the exercise program.

Study Makes a Big Impact on the Unified Parkinson's Disease Rating Scale

The motor symptoms of the cycle control group, as measured using the Movement Disorders Society-Unified Parkinson's Disease Rating Scale (MDS-UPDRS), stabilized during the exercise period in the cycling group, whereas the control group that merely did stretching exercises declined over time, as one would normally expect with a progressive condition like PD. An article by *Science Daily* reported that the Park-in-Shape study was a large, at-home, double-blind study, which showed that patients in the early stages of Parkinson's disease who exercised three times a week for six months experienced improved motor symptoms from exercise comparable to the effect of conventional Parkinson's medication. The news outlet went on to interview PhD candidate Nicolien van der Kolk, who said, "After the study, the cycling patients had a significantly better cardiovascular fitness, which has many obvious advantages. The motor disability of the cycling group was also significantly better: according to the gold standard (the MDS-UPDRS score), the cycling group scored on average 4.2 points lower than the control group" (Radboud, "Exercising").

Professor Bloem, the principal investigator, said, "This study is very important. We can now start researching whether much more long-term cycling can also slow the disease progression. Also, this new 'exergam-

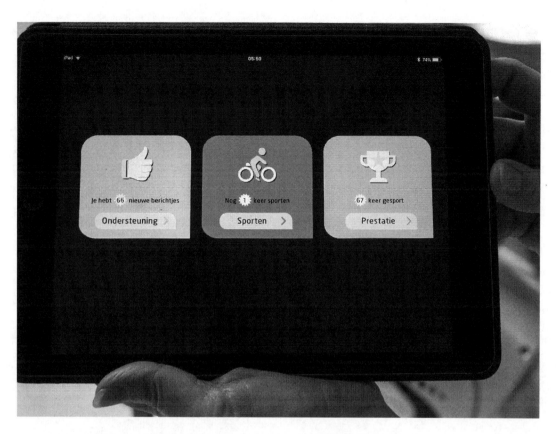

The aerobic-exercise group had stationary bikes with gaming equipment called "exergaming"—a form of motivation. The exergaming equipment also gave the participant feedback on their rides and encouragement.

ing' approach that we have developed is very suitable to achieve long-term improvements in exercise behavior for patients with a range of other disorders that could also benefit from regular exercise" (Radboud, "Exercising").

Subset of Study Group Participated in Phase II of Park-in-Shape Study

A subset of participants from the *Park-in-Shape study* joined in Phase II of Park-in-Shape titled *Aerobic Exercise Alters Brain Function and Structure in Parkinson's Disease: A Randomized Controlled Trial* (Johansson et al. 2022). Twenty-five were in the aerobic exercise group, and thirty-one were in the active control group (stretching). This study "tested the hypothesis that aerobic exercise slows the natural circuit-level progression of PD" (Johansson et al. 2). The groups underwent resting-state functional and structural magnetic resonance imaging (MRI) at the beginning and at the six-month mark. The researchers were looking at how aerobic exercise influences brain function and structure. Specifically, they looked at sections of the brain involved in motor and cognitive functions affected by PD. The nerves involving sensor motor function, known as the sensorimotor network, are part of the eventual motor loss in PD (Johansson et al. 209).

Chapter 2

Part of the Brain Involved with Motor Function Did Not Show Brain Atrophy after High-Intensity Aerobic Exercise

Healthy individuals' cortical sensorimotor regions generally communicate with the posterior putamen (a large dark lateral part of the basal ganglion). PWPD rely more on the anterior putamen. Since the putamen is a brain region involved in motor function control, and its posterior portion is heavily affected in early PD, the subset study results were significant. The results showed that in the higher-intensity aerobic exercise group, their brains did not show atrophy. However, the brains of the stretching group did show atrophy. Even more impressive, new connections formed between the diseased basal ganglia and the healthy cortex in the high-intensity group (Johansson et al. 213-215).

Park-in-Shape Phase II Found Exercise Stimulates Neuroplasticity in the Brain

The *Park-in-Shape Phase II study* focused on how aerobic exercise influences disease-related changes in the corticostriatal sensorimotor network. The network is involved in the development of motor loss in PD. The study found that "Brain atrophy is a primary pathological hallmark of PD and is associated with progression of motor and cognitive symptoms. Here, brain atrophy worsened over time in the stretching group . . . Aerobic exercise improved cognitive control, as indexed by an oculomotor task known to be sensitive to executive deficits in PD" (Johansson et al. 214).

> *Parts of the brain that were damaged by Parkinson's disease, called the basal ganglia, made new connections to the healthy brain cortex—which is where you plan all your movements. This is wholly exciting because the brain was reshaping itself in a beneficial way under the influence of exercise. Really, those findings should motivate every person with Parkinson's to the bone, you know, to the bone to start exercising faithfully.*

- Professor Bastiaan R. Bloem

I asked Professor Bloem to explain why this study was important. He said, "The reason our Park-in-Shape Study was so exciting is that the people who were faithful to exercise three times a week for 30 minutes at 80% maximum heart rate stabilized their motor symptoms. So, they did not decline over time. We also saw some improvement in cognitive functions. But more importantly, we also did brain scans in both the exercise group and the stretching control groups. We noted that the brain was shrinking a little bit over time, which is what you would expect in all of us. However, that shrinkage was stopped in the exercise group. Moreover, the parts of the brain that were damaged by Parkinson's disease, called the basal ganglia, made new connections to the healthy brain cortex—which is where you plan all your movements. This is wholly exciting because the brain was reshaping itself in a beneficial way under the influence of exercise. Really, those findings should motivate every person with Parkinson's to the bone, you know, to the bone to start exercising faithfully." These findings by Professor Bloem and his colleagues should inspire everyone with PD to start exercising right away.

Dr Alberts' Latest U.S. PD Cycle Study Is Expected to Come Back with the Best Data Ever

In 2019, Dr. Alberts received a $3-million-dollar grant from the National Institute of Neurological Disorders and Stroke (NINDS) to conduct a five-year, multi-site clinical trial: *Effectiveness of a Long-Term, Home-Based Aerobic Exercise Intervention on Slowing the Progression of Parkinson Disease: Design of the Cyclical Lower Extremity Exercise for Parkinson Disease (CYCLE-II) Study*. The study is researching the long-term effects of high-intensity aerobic exercise, in home-based settings, on slowing the progression of PD. Dr. Alberts said, "This will be one of the largest groups to have such a fine assessment of cognitive functions, motor functions, and activity level. And the importance of this is the fact that all these people, regardless of what group they are in, are pioneers in PD research. They are providing us with very valuable information about the progression of the disease. If you look in the literature, the progression of the disease ranges from two points to eleven points on the UPDRS. That's a problem when you start thinking about disease progression and altering disease progression and trying to measure it appropriately. I think the research we receive from CYCLE II will provide some of the best data to measure disease progression."

CHAPTER 3

The Cost of Inactivity for Someone with PD Is Worsening Symptoms and a Shorter Life Span

"Research tells us that an exercise prescription is one of the best ways to
slow Parkinson's progression and retain physical and even cognitive function,
as well as facilitate other functions, like sleep, digestion, and mood.
If your doctor gave you a prescriptive pill that could improve all those areas,
without downsides, you'd fill that in a heartbeat."

- Davis Phinney, founder of
the Davis Phinney Foundation for Parkinson's

A Rude Awakening . . . The COVID-19 Pandemic

The first indoor Neuro Cycle ride, back after a delay caused by the COVID-19 pandemic (which kept riders out of the cycle studio for three months), was worse than when we started riding for the first time years prior. It was unexpected and jolting.

Clients I had worked with for years displayed symptoms I had never seen before. It took my breath away. And riding the bike again took all our breaths away. It was like climbing the biggest hill we had ever encountered. Gone was the optimal 80-85 RPM they had worked hard to achieve. Instead, watts (strength output) plummeted. How was this possible in such a short amount of time? Most heart-wrenching was to see my clients struggling with symptoms they didn't have before COVID-19 showed up at our door.

"When COVID-19 hit, I thought, 'This is only going to last a short while,' and then after several months I thought, 'I need to do something fast, I'm losing ground here,'" explained my client, Sandy Trent. "So, I joined Zoom classes and started walking, but it still wasn't enough. On Mother's Day, I fell and no matter what position I tried, I couldn't get up. I was stuck on the ground for six hours. Lying there, unable to get myself up for the first time in years, I began thinking about my choices. I could either go to a nursing home and lose more movement and brain function, and risk getting the deadly virus. Or I could choose to go back to the workout center, which had taken all the necessary precautions to make me feel safe. And, boy, my first cycle ride was incredibly difficult. I had gone down to 50 RPM and 25 watts. But I improved every day and worked my way back up."

COVID-19 Reminded Us What We Already Knew Was True about PD . . . Rapid Deterioration Occurs With Inactivity

COVID-19 disrupted the lives of many people in so many ways. The Michael J. Fox Foundation's *The Effect of the COVID-19 Pandemic on People with Parkinson's Disease Study* (Brown et al. 1365–1377) in 2020, revealed crucial information regarding PD patients. Of the 5,429 people with PD and 1,452 without PD who responded to a survey as part of the study, "COVID-19 diagnoses were reported by 51 people with and 26 without PD. Complications were more frequent in people with longer PD duration. People with PD and COVID-19 experienced new or worsening motor (63%) and nonmotor (75%) symptoms. People with PD not diagnosed with COVID-19 reported disrupted medical care (64%), exercise (21%), and social activities (57%), and worsened motor (43%) and non-motor (52%) symptoms." Non-motor symptoms included mood issues, digestive problems, pain, and fatigue (Brown et al. 1365).

PWPD Suffered New or Worsening Symptoms from Inactivity as if They Had Gotten the COVID-19 Virus

Even more incredible is that the number of PD people who didn't get COVID-19 nevertheless suffered from the pandemic experience as if they had gotten the virus. "For people with PD without COVID-19, disruptions were frequent in PD-related medical care (64%), essential daily activities (35%), exercise (21%), and social activity (57%), and contributed to worsening of motor and non-motor symptoms, especially in specific at-risk groups" (Brown et al. 1374). So the statistics show that although these PWPD didn't get COVID-19, their motor and non-motor symptoms got worse by a whopping 43% and 52%, respectively, because their lives and exercise routines were interrupted.

Three Months of Missed Exercise Left Everyone Hurting

Before COVID-19, my client Bill Brown (age 80), a retired marketing executive, attended my PD cycling class four days a week. He also worked with a personal trainer and did progressive strength training two days a week. He rarely missed a class unless the fish were biting and then the fly fisherman in him couldn't help but take the weekend off to do what he loved.

During the three-month COVID-19 lockdown he tried everything to keep his activity level up while away from his PD classes. He walked two miles daily with his wife and did online workout classes, but he quickly found that it wasn't the same as his PD-specific classes that were designed to help clients achieve goals based on science.

"The first (cycle) ride, back after missing three months due to COVID-19, was brutal," commented Bill, "and walking two miles a day didn't even begin to cut it for keeping my symptoms at bay. I will say that when I first stopped neuro-cycling, I felt the benefits of high-intensity bike classes for about four weeks. But then the benefits and symptom relief dropped incredibly fast. Without cycling, I noticed my balance getting rapidly worse. And I had gotten to such a great place through cycling. I was hitting up to 80-90 RPM on my metric assessment rides with my watts up in the 130 range. After COVID, it was 50 RPM, and the watts were so low. I lost so much ground so fast that I just couldn't believe it. It was tough building back up."

If You Have PD and Don't Exercise, Your Risk of Early Death Is Higher

Without exercise, PD progresses faster. Professor Bloem stated the following at the *2020 Parkinson's Academy's Webinar, Exercise in Parkinson's during COVID-19*: "The adverse effects of inactivity include cardiovascular disease, osteoporosis, insomnia, cognitive decline, depression, and constipation . . . All

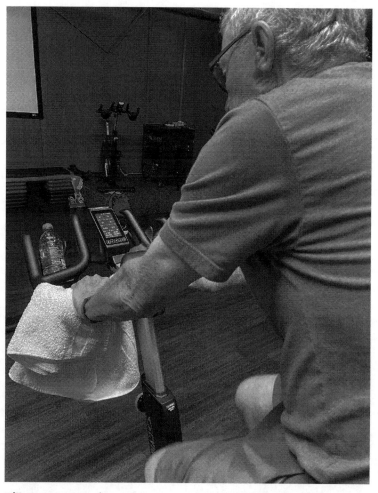

Bill Brown experienced extreme changes in symptoms after the COVID-19 lockdown due to his inability to work at high-intensity levels.

these are risk factors when you have Parkinson's; so if you are both inactive and have Parkinson's, your risk of early mortality is higher" (Bloem "Exercise").

As we learned in Chapter 2, for far too long, people diagnosed with PD were sent home and told to sit. And yet today, many PWPD follow this practice of inactivity, not realizing this is the worst thing they can do. "Inactivity in PD was associated with worse walking performance, more disability in daily life, and greater disease severity" (Van Nimwegen et al. 2219).

A 2021 COVID-19 impact study explained the effects of inactivity and stress on PWPD. "COVID-19 induced the exacerbation of disease-specific symptoms in Parkinson's disease. It has been stated that worsened symptoms were slowness, stiffness/rigidity, tremor, gait, freezing of gait, speech, easy fatigability, pain, sleep disorders, concentration, feeling stressed, anxiety–depression, constipation, and forgetfulness during the outbreak" (Balci et al. 175).

> *The adverse effects of inactivity include cardiovascular disease, osteoporosis, insomnia, cognitive decline, depression, and constipation . . . all these are risk factors when you have Parkinson's; so if you are both inactive and have Parkinson's, your risk of early mortality is higher.*
>
> **- Professor Bastiaan R. Bloem**

As you can see from my clients who took only three months off during COVID-19, climbing back from losing the strength and aerobic capability they had spent years building was challenging. But they did get it back—one day at a time. And you can, too. You just have to start. What's important to realize is that losses apply to everyday inactivity. We don't need a pandemic for these losses to happen. They are happening each day that focused, purposeful movement is not occurring.

Why Daily Exercise Is Critical for PWPD

Professor Bloem says, "Daily exercise is critical for those living with Parkinson's because:

- Exercise helps your heart, brain, bone density, lungs, and more.
- Exercise may prevent Parkinson's.
- If you have Parkinson's, exercise works like medication. It is continually proven by research that exercise suppresses symptoms of Parkinson's.
- It is currently believed that if anything can slow the progression of Parkinson's, it's regular exercise" (Bloem "Exercise").

Eight Life-Changing Results from Consistent, High-Intensity Exercise

Here is the best news. Eight life-changing positive effects of high-intensity exercise on the brain have been documented in a review (Mahalakshmi et al. 2020) on exercise and neuroprotective mechanisms (see more details on this review in Chapter 4).

1. Exercise improves mood and sleep.
2. Exercise reduces stress and anxiety (Dauwan et al. qtd. in Mahalakshmi et al. 2).
3. Exercise reduces insulin resistance. For people with PD, insulin resistance causes a faster progression of motor symptoms—tremors, rigidity, bradykinesia and so forth.
4. Exercise reduces inflammation. Chronic inflammation contributes to the condition and progression of PD. The reduction of inflammation is a phenomenal benefit in helping to slow the progression of the disease (Barrientos et al. qtd. in Mahalakshmi et al. 1) (Mee-Inta et al. qtd. in Mahalakshmi et al. 4).
5. Exercise stimulates growth and releases growth factors—naturally occurring substances capable of stimulating cellular growth, proliferation, and cellular differentiation—offering a promising approach to neuroprotection and neurorestoration for PD. However, using growth factor drug replacement has been found too difficult and insufficiently safe for treating PD. Fortunately, exercise is being shown to safely release growth factors naturally (Mahalakshmi et al. 1).
6. Exercise stimulates the growth of new blood vessels (Paillard as qtd. in Mahalakshmi et al. 6). A 2022 pilot trial (Inacio "Pilot"), studying how a biological compound stimulates new blood vessel growth in the brain for people with PD, theorizes that restoring blood flow with new blood vessels—known as angiogenesis—can slow and even reverse the progression of PD. However, like growth factors, it is still not known how safe such compounds are for humans. Until current studies of the compounds are completed, exercise is a safe way to achieve the growth of new blood vessels.
7. Exercise improves memory and learning (rewiring and neuroplasticity; see more in Chapter 4) (Philips et al. qtd. in Mahalakshmi et al. 9).
8. Exercise preserves brain cells' overall health, abundance, and survival (neuronal survival, see more in Chapter 4) (Mahalakshmi et al. 8).

These eight life-changing results offer enormous benefit for PWPD, and with no side effects. There are other benefits as well. Exercise helps with depression and anxiety. It improves the integrity and density of white matter in the brain, which speeds up our ability to make neural connections. These benefits enhance the quality of life—which is essential not just for PWPD but for everyone.

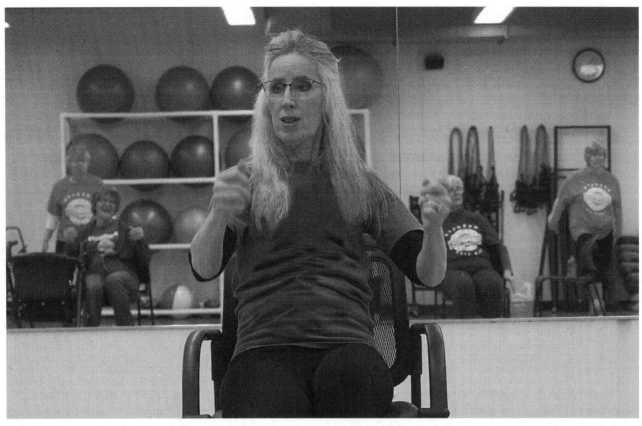

You can get a great cardio workout in a chair. In this photo you see some people in chairs, Jane Collison demonstrating, and some people standing. People who use canes and walkers come to classes. They ride bikes, hit the bag for boxing, and perform their resistance training. There are always ways to make it work.

Photo by Laraine Davis

Hitting 80% of Max Heart Rate Isn't as Hard as You Think

I know what you are thinking: there is no way you can do "high-intensity or hit 80%—85% of maximum heart rate." But I'm here to tell you, "YES! You can!" And it's easier than you think. When I am speaking to a group of people with PD, they get nervous when they keep hearing me say that they will have to do "high-intensity" workouts to stabilize or get positive results for their PD symptoms, or to help slow disease progression. That is when I let them in on a little secret. I explain, "It's harder for an in-shape person to hit 80% of maximum heart rate (or 7–8 on a 10-perceived-exertion scale—a measure of how hard you are working based on your own physical sensations) than someone who hasn't been working out at all." They laugh, with a sigh of relief.

And here is the reason why it isn't as hard as you'd expect. If you have not been working out for a while, then marching briskly in place and pumping your arms will quickly make you feel breathless—an indication that you are close to that 80% heart-rate zone we want you to hit. On the other hand, someone in shape would have to run in place pumping their arms overhead to get to that same breathless level. It's takes a highly individualized amount of effort to hit that high-intensity target.

As Your Aerobic Endurance Base Improves Over Time, You Will Have to Increase Your Effort

Your aerobic endurance base changes over time as you get in better cardiovascular shape, which means you will have to increase your effort as you continue to improve. But the process is slow and unique to each person. As you progress, one quick measure to see if you are in the correct aerobic range is that you are feeling winded, sweating, or both. Chapter 7 will talk about finding your heart rate or using a "Perceived Exertion Chart" if heart-rate zones don't work for you.

You Can Do This . . . Many People with Extraordinary Physical Challenges Are Already Exercising

When people tell me they will never be able to exercise at higher intensity levels, I introduce them to Sandy, whom I mentioned earlier. Sandy is completely paralyzed on one side of her body, yet she worked her way up to be able to hit high-intensity levels on the bike and in cardio classes. I have people who use canes and walkers that come to class and ride bikes, work from chairs, and hit the boxing bag, or perform aerobic classes in a chair. People will strength-train with walkers, wheelchairs, or a cane, which they put down after they sit, and then start their workout. There are ways to make exercise work for anyone. There is truth to the saying, "Where there's a will, there's a way." You may just need an exercise professional who works with PWPD, or a physical therapist, depending on your situation, to help you figure out how to make it work for you.

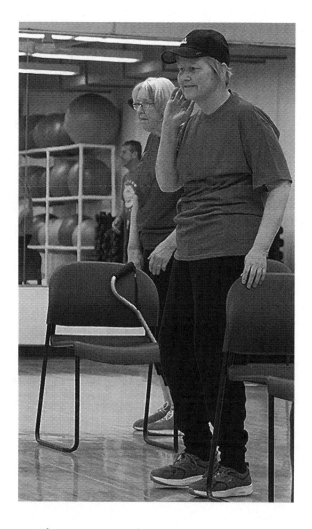

In this photo are Juli Aufdenkamp (wearing the baseball cap—you will read about her in the next chapter), Sandy Trent, and Joe Hingl. Juli is blind and is following me in the class through verbal cues. Next to her is Sandy Trent, who is working with one side of her body paralyzed. You may notice that they both keep a chair next to them in case they need to grab it for support. I like to remind any new PWPD wanting to try a neuro or PD class, but is having reservations, "Anything is possible. Just look at what Sandy and Juli are doing!"

Photo by Laraine Davis

Chapter 3

CHAPTER 4

The Science Behind PD Exercise

"My research study was written about in *Annals of Neurology* (Johansson 203-216)—
one of the elite journals in our field. The study showed that when people cycled on a home
trainer for 30 to 45 minutes three times a week, compared to a control group merely
doing stretching exercises, that brain atrophy, the shrinking of the brain
which is happening in all of us, was stopped. And the brain in the exercise group
started to make new functional connections between the diseased basal ganglia,
and the healthy cortex. So, brain plasticity is induced by exercise in people with Parkinson's.
Boy, if that doesn't stimulate all of you to hop on your bicycle, or jump on your treadmill
to start exercising, then I've done something wrong in my talk today."

- Bastiaan R. Bloem, MD, PhD, FRCPE

Why the Science Behind PD Exercise Makes So Much Sense to Me

One of my PD clients, Kay Arvidson, visited her internist for a routine checkup. She had noticed a tremor in her hand. Her doctor ordered a brain scan, which put Kay into a state of panic because she was convinced she had brain cancer. Kay was a breast cancer survivor and immediately thought the cancer was back. She barely remembers the process of having the scan done because she was still in utter shock. She just "knew" it was cancer.

She was sent to a neurologist who told her at her examination, "You have Parkinson's." She just stared in disbelief. Kay finally said to the neurologist blankly, "I don't even know what that is." She vaguely remembers the doctor mentioning "exercise" and saying "Go to a PD website and conference to learn more about the disease."

Kay Experienced PD Symptoms She Didn't Expect

Kay's tremor quickly got worse. Before she knew it, she also had dyskinesia (uncontrollable body movements) and dystonia (muscles contracting involuntarily), both of which can be incredibly painful. Both symptoms can also cause repetitive and twisting movements. Her medication was increased, and so, feeling better, Kay started to attend a Rock Steady Boxing class in the hopes of slowing her symptoms and disease progression down. However, her symptoms were increasing at such a rate that, in 2021, she became a candidate for Deep Brain Stimulation (DBS) surgery, which involves the implantation of a device to send electrical signals to the brain.

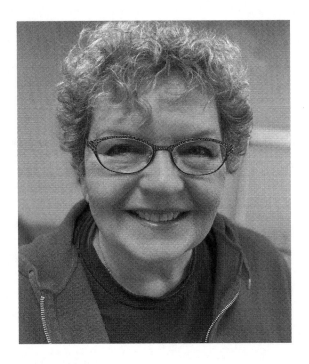

Kay Arvidson learned first-hand that PD science-based exercise is her secret weapon against her fight with PD.

DBS Surgery Did Wonders to Help Kay with Her Symptoms

A 2020 study of *DBS surgery for PD* shows that "The mean (range) age at surgery was 60 (42–78) years, and the duration of disease was 13 (5–25) years" (Thomsen et al. 789). Kay had severe enough symptoms to warrant DBS surgery four years after her diagnosis. In April of 2021, after delays caused by the COVID-19 pandemic, she finally got into the hospital for DBS treatment. Kay responded well to the surgery, and her symptoms improved significantly. However, the COVID lockdown did not help her situation. As we learned in Chapter 3, it doesn't take long to lose significant gains, even from surgery. Kay was not an exception to the PD inactivity rule—no one is.

Kay Realized That Knowledge Is Power and We All have More Than We Realize

Kay realized that medicine and surgery help, but they don't slow PD's fast-moving progress that spirals downward both in motor and non-motor symptoms. In October of 2021, she heard my presentation, *How to Exercise to Reduce Parkinson's Symptoms—The Science Behind Parkinson's Exercise*, at the 2021 American Parkinson's Disease Association (APDA) Iowa Chapter Optimism Conference.

Kay signed up to become part of my Neuro-Wellness Program the next day. Kay shares how this information deeply affected her. "I've always believed that knowledge is power. I discovered that we don't realize how much power we have. There are times when we have more ability than we think we can exert, which I discovered when I learned about the science behind PD exercise. I can affect my symptoms and help slow my disease progression by choosing the right PD exercise at the right time and performing it the right way.

"I also realized this would change over time as my PD changes, but I have the power to control my destiny through exercise. I want to control my PD to the best of my ability. And that is why the science behind PD exercise makes so much sense to me."

Exercise Programs Offer Support and Camaraderie

Kay and I sat down and figured out her PD Exercise Cocktail Plan™ (see Chapter 5), which initially started with two weekly cycling classes and two Total Health Works' (THW) Total Parkinson's classes. Kay's cocktail of choice is a screwdriver, and her PD exercise battle cry is, "Screw You, Parkinson's!"

Kay shared, "I was equally amazed by the ease I experienced starting to exercise in this program and the warmth and camaraderie I found with this exercise group. I enjoy the THW's Total Parkinson's class and seeing my movement improve. I was scared to try cycling but was surprised to find it was fun. I feel a big difference in my motor skills immediately after cycling. I was surprised by the positive change in how I felt and moved."

Since Finding PD Exercise, Her Entire Life Has Changed for the Better

Since Kay began exercising, we have added treadmill and progressive strength training to her PD program plan. In fact, her favorite workout is progressive strength training with instability—where she may put one foot on a balance pad while doing bicep curls (see Chapter 10). She can really feel her brain activate during this exercise.

For the past year, Kay has been managing her symptoms beautifully and has found that the more she exercises consistently, the better she feels. Her life has completely changed into a new routine. She said, "I can tell immediately after a cycling class that I have impacted my illness. My movement has dramatically improved. I feel good. I don't sit around or watch TV anymore. I'm either working on my PD exercise or my PD volunteer work. I love it, and my life is fulfilled."

What Is Parkinson's Doing to the Brain?

For most people, PD is a slow, progressive, degenerative disease. Over time, a loss of cells that produce dopamine occurs in the substantia nigra pars compacta—the part of your brain that controls your body's movements. In addition, dopamine depletion occurs in the striatum, a neural circuit responsible for voluntary movement (Zhang 108). Lack of dopamine helps to explain what is creating the motor symptoms—bradykinesia, tremor, rigidity, slow movement, freezing, and dystonia.

Lewy Bodies Are Unusual Clumps of a Protein That kills Dopamine in the Brain

Many of the brain cells of PWPD contain Lewy bodies. Lewy bodies are an aggregation of unusual clumps of alpha-synuclein protein (Reynolds, "Tracking"). These clumps of an alpha-synuclein protein are what kill dopamine in the brain, and the collection of Lewy bodies contributes to the progression of PD.

International Review finds Exercise Works Across Neurodegenerative Diseases

In Chapter 3, I said I would go into more detail about the 2020 review titled *Possible Neuroprotective Mechanisms of Physical Exercise in Neurodegeneration*. The scientists looked at previous research on exercise and its neuroprotective capabilities resulting in potential attenuation of neurodegeneration (or slowing disease progression by halting neuron loss) (Mahalakshmi et al. 1). The review also looked at how physical exercise improved physical performance, mental status, general health, and well-being in people with neurological diseases. The authors explained that exercise created many mechanisms at the individuals' cellular and molecular levels. Within these mechanisms are "direct participants" or so-called "signaling mechanisms"—proteins, such as brain-derived neurotrophic factors, hormones like irisin (also known as "the exercise hormone"), and neurotransmitters like dopamine (Mahalakshmi et al. 10).

High-Intensity Exercise Might Help to Preserve Neurons in the Brain and Enable It to Relearn Things That PD Has Taken Away

The review explained that high-intensity physical exercise helps preserve neurons and promotes neuroplasticity—how the brain rewires to change for the better in PD. The review states, "A meta-analysis prepared evidence on the safety and efficacy of physical exercise as an additional therapeutic intervention for the quality of life, cognition, and depressive symptoms across six chronic brain disorders" (Mahalakshmi et al. 10). The review also suggested that exercising is superior to usual treatment in improving quality of life, depressive symptoms, attention, working memory, and psychomotor speed (Dauwan qtd. at Mahalakshmi et al. 2).

High-Intensity Exercise May Slow PD Progression by Avoiding Protein Buildup in the Brain

The review defines how high-intensity activities like biking, running, and moving with intensity activate these "signaling mechanisms." It is through (exercise's) higher intensities that the most benefits are derived. The review stated, "Neurotrophins like BDNF [brain-derived neurotropic factor], hormones like irisin, and neurotransmitters like dopamine are direct participants in these mechanisms. Considering its effect among PD patients, it improves gait, balance, cognition, along with a slowing down progression of the disease by avoiding protein aggregation in the brain" (Mahalakshmi et al. 10). A 2018 review titled *Aerobic Exercise: Evidence for a Direct Brain Effect to Slow Parkinson Disease Progression* proposes that exercise creates the mechanisms that for a neural response that may help slow disease progression for those with PD (Ahlskog et al. 366-367).

How Exercise Rewires the Brain for Change

Neuroplasticity is a word PWPD often hear regarding PD and other neurological diseases. "Neuroplasticity refers to the brain's ability to undergo structural and functional reorganization in response to learning or experience . . . the 'use it or lose it' also applies to neuroplasticity, where a lack of activity between neurons within a circuit leads to a decrease in the strength of connection between these neurons" (Liebert qtd. Pickersgill et al. 2022. 1).

There have been relatively few PWPD studies regarding neuroplasticity, though things do look promising going forward. A review titled *Exercise-Induced Neuroplasticity in Parkinson's Disease: A Metasynthesis of the Literature* stated that, "Our results indicate that various forms of physical exercise may lead to changes in various markers of neuroplasticity. A narrative synthesis suggests that brain function and structure can be altered in a positive direction after an exercise period" (Johansson et al. 1).

That is why, for instance, a THW's Total Parkinson's class will incorporate short, high-intensity rounds of cardio intervals followed by PD-specific exercises like memory work, large-amplitude walking, or balance exercises. These exercises are an opportunity to work on capabilities that PD has taken away. However, neuroplasticity and brain changes to help improve PD symptoms do not just happen with random, unstructured exercise. To achieve this, you must hit the MHR intensity levels determined by the scientists' research described in this book.

Brain-Derived Neurotrophic Factor (BDNF) Is a Gamechanger for PD

To kickstart BDNF levels in the brain, you must first elevate your heart rate. Second, the heart rate must stay elevated for an extended period. Third, and most important, is consistency. BDNF is generous in that it multiplies quickly but it doesn't sit around forever. To make the protein do its magic, you must perform high-intensity aerobic endurance workouts at least three times a week.

A 2020 PD cycling study in Bogotá, Colombia titled *Effect of a High-Intensity Tandem Bicycle Exercise Program on Clinical Severity, Functional Magnetic Resonance Imaging, and Plasma Biomarkers in Parkinson's Disease* (Segura et al. 1), had two groups of PWPD. The intervention group (IG) rode on the back seats of tandem bikes at 80% of MHR three times a week for sixteen weeks. The control group (CG) did not ride at the IG MHR level (Segura 1). Statistics from the report showed that the "Mean Unified Parkinson's Disease Rating Scale (UPDRS) went down by 5.7 points in the IG and showed a small 0.9-point increase in the CG (p = 0.11)" (Segura et al. 1). What was quite remarkable was that the BDNF levels in the IG increased more than ten-fold, while the CG group decreased its BDNF levels.

Hormones and Neurotrophic Factors Must Cross the Blood Brain Barrier to Effect Changes

Another important factor is the blood-brain barrier (BBB). The BBB's main job is to stop unwanted substances that could injure the brain from reaching that organ. However, the BBB does allow some materials—such as [or including] irisin and BDNF—to cross, which is vital in helping PD.

Why All This Science Is Important to You

Finally, consider these three research highlights. A 2021 study titled *Aerobic Exercise Alters Brain Function and Structure in Parkinson's Disease: A Randomized Controlled Trial* (Johansson et al.), printed in the *Annals of Neurology*, provided something scientists have been waiting a very long time for—concrete evidence in human studies that intense aerobic exercise stimulates neuroplasticity in the brain (214).

An original investigation titled *Association of Levels of Physical Activity with Risk of Parkinson Disease—A Systematic Review and Meta-Analysis* looked at eight prospective studies totaling 544,336 participants included 2,192 patients with PD (Fang et al. 4). The investigation found that "this meta-analysis is the largest and most comprehensive evaluation of the dose-response relationship between physical activity and the risk of PD in the general population. Using data extracted from prospective studies, our pooled analysis of more than half a million adults revealed that higher levels of physical activity—particularly moderate to vigorous activity—are associated with a lower risk of developing PD" (Fang et al. 6).

According to a peer-reviewed paper titled *The Universal Prescription for Parkinson's Disease: Exercise* (Alberts and Rosenfeldt 2020), "There is evidence that aerobic exercise results in structural and functional CNS [central nervous system] changes in healthy older adults and PWPD. After a single bout of high intensity forced-exercise, functional MRI data indicated altered CNS patterns of activation in the primary motor cortex, supplementary motor area, thalamus, globus pallidus, and putamen in PWPD, similar to patterns seen following levodopa administration. In a subsequent study, individuals pedaling at a higher cadence during an eight-week stationary cycling intervention exhibited greater increases in cortico-subcortical connectivity during task performance compared to those who pedaled slower. Importantly, results from these and other human imaging and mechanistic studies indicate that aerobic exercise is capable of improving CNS function, supporting that exercise is medicine for PD" (Alberts and Rosenfeldt S22-S23).

The idea seems almost too simple; that exercise, something we do every day of our lives—moving, using our joints and muscles purposefully in a way prescribed in this book—can be a key to holding at bay, and perhaps someday reversing, one of the cruelest diseases that afflicts the human race. Yet, in recent years, hundreds of top research scientists throughout the world have spent thousands of hours investigating and validating this link. The overwhelming evidence, as briefly summarized in this chapter, is that . . . it works! High-intensity exercise, performed in individually tailored plans and carried out in conjunction with trained professionals, can potentially turn the tide against PD.

CHAPTER 5

PD Exercise Cocktail Plans™ and Recommendations

"Do not confuse my bad days as a sign of weakness.
Those are actually the days I'm fighting my hardest."

- Author Unknown

The Power of Exercise Can Impact Someone's Entire Family in a Way They Never Expected

My client Joe Hingl (age 55), a retired salesman, came to his first neuro-cycle class after his wife, Kelly, told him about the Neuro-Wellness Program. He had been diagnosed with multiple sclerosis (MS) four years previously and came to class walking with a cane. He quickly became the life of the party and made everyone in class laugh and smile with his amazing sense of humor. He also worked extremely hard in class—cycling three times a week and participating in a Total HealthWorks' (THW) Total Parkinson's class two times a week.

Four months after he began attending classes, Joe no longer needed his cane. He could walk without it again. He commented, "I have benefited from classes both mentally and physically. It is very important to have our support group. It helps to know other people have challenges to overcome and we are not alone in our daily struggles. I know I must work hard every day to maintain and delay the progression of my illness."

Later, we adjusted Joe's Exercise Cocktail Plan™ (see below about building PD Exercise Cocktail Plan™s), which he named his "Old Fashioned Make It Happen." Joe was happy with the brain and body class because it heavily emphasizes balance work. He was feeling great and making tremendous strides. Joe also wanted to try a neuro-aqua class, which turned out to be eye-opening for him. It gave him freedom of movement he didn't feel on land. It helped both his aerobic performance and his balance. Later he added progressive strength training to his plan, which was a good complement to his aerobic endurance work.

The most heart-warming part of Joe's story is that, months later, he could walk his daughter down the aisle at her wedding without using his cane. This would never have been possible if he hadn't executed his Exercise Cocktail Plan™. This is the kind of life-changing result that I am incredibly happy to witness. Joe said, "I think everyone has challenges to overcome, and if you look around, there is always someone else climbing a more giant mountain than you are—those are the people we can look up to for inspiration. So, it's enriching to set goals and try to meet them. The goal might be to exercise for thirty minutes, or maybe it's a mileage goal to make during a cycle class. Some days it's to get out of bed in the morning. Set goals and meet them. I feel great when I have accomplished my weekly goals because everything I do here in the gym helps me delay my illness or at least maintain it. Neurodegenerative diseases don't take any breaks. They are with us when we wake up, all through the day, and while we sleep. It's up to me to diligently beat it back every day. And I exercise daily for my family and myself."

Having a Daily Exercise Support Group Is Important for Success

PD can be depressing and brutal to tackle daily, so, belonging to a Neuro-Wellness Program with an exercise support group to help each other daily does more for PWPD than I can describe. But Joe Hingl, who you just read about, would tell you firsthand how necessary it is. I asked Joe, "If you were going to describe to someone who was apprehensive about trying a neuro-exercise program, what kind of advice would you give that person?"

Joe answered, "We are hesitant to put ourselves out there and go exercise with a new group of people. Perhaps we all have challenges we are overcoming, and we don't want others to see those challenges. But whether they are internal or external, everyone has challenges. By working out with a group, we can get past those and support one another. We laugh and have fun, and it becomes positive reinforcement when we realize we are not alone in our daily struggles."

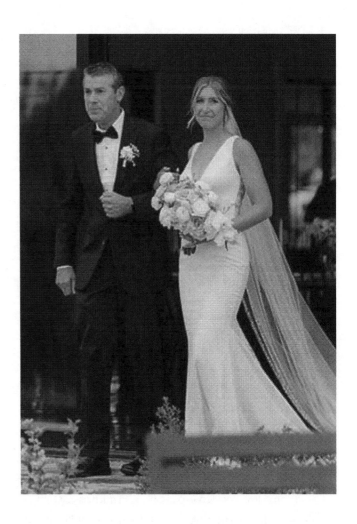

Because Joe Hingl implemented his "Old Fashioned Make It Happen" Cocktail Exercise Plan™, he could walk his daughter, Grace, down the aisle without using a cane, which means the world to him and his family.

PWPD Need a Personal Cocktail to Fuel Their Journey

I devised a fun way to categorize my client's PD exercise workout program plans. I refer to them as exercise "cocktails." The plans are highly individualized, just like their beverages of choice. And people love coming up with names for exercise cocktails. They think of their favorite drink and add a fun phrase of motivation—like Joe Johll's "Margarita Fight Back Plan."

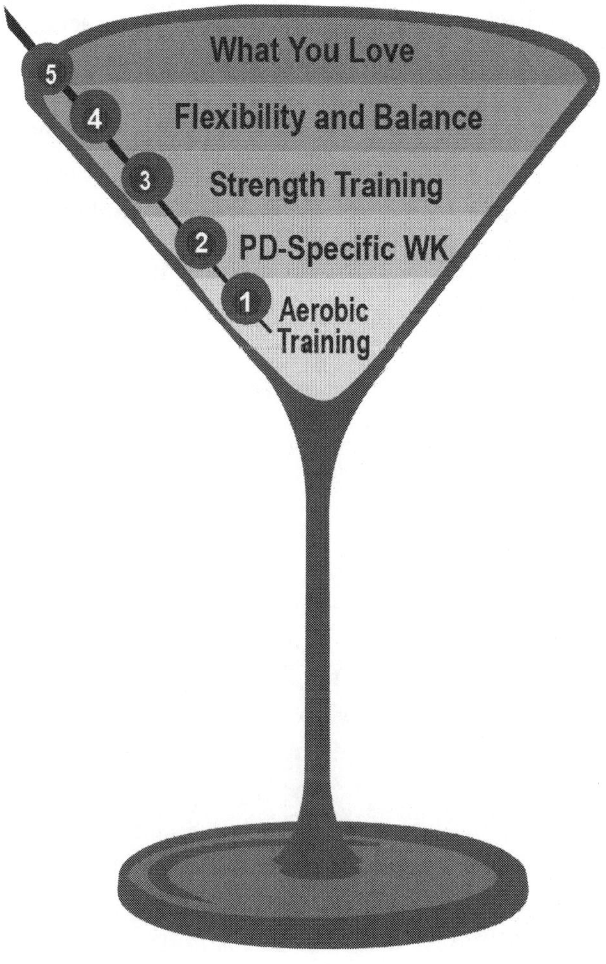

Figure 2: PD Exercise Cocktail Plan™

Building a PD Exercise Cocktail Plan™. First, make sure you have fun creating a name for your cocktail to motivate you. The steps in the graphic show what takes place in building a PD Exercise Cocktail Plan™. Level 1 is the most critical layer. You will start with Level 1 and add additional levels from 1–4, depending upon the stage of disease, motivation, and goals. Level 5 is doing what you love—the "olive or maraschino cherry" on top, making it complete.

When building a PD Exercise Cocktail Plan™, I first determine the PWPD's balance, walking, rotation, and movement abilities through formal assessments. After assessments, I find out what they want to work on, symptom-wise, and what exercise they like. We figure out what cardio or strength program will work best for them. And we discuss how to tackle symptoms as they appear or change throughout their PD journey. Then, I perform monthly assessments to see where they are in their progress.

If they struggle most with multiple PD-specific symptoms, I may suggest a THW's Total Parkinson's class or Tai Chi for balance. If they need to improve their gait, depending on the severity of their issues, I will send them to a PD physical therapist for gait training. If they want to work on tremors and cognition, then I recommend progressive strength training (assigning them a personal trainer who is experienced working with PWPD), and they can also try different class options—Rock Steady Boxing (RSB), PWR!Moves© online class, Movement-Revolution online class, for example—with strength training available or incorporated into the class, to see what works for them.

My goal is that they find what they love to do so that they will continue exercising. It is essential to build up the layers of the cocktail over time, depending on the disease stage, the person's level of fitness, what each individual likes to do, and their goals.

Build Your PD Exercise Cocktail Plan™ With a Physical Therapist or Exercise Professional Who Works with PWPD

Let's build an example PD Exercise Cocktail Plan™ from scratch. Before getting to the different levels, first choose your favorite beverage and add a motivating tagline. It doesn't matter if you don't drink anymore. Think of a drink you used to like or something non-alcoholic that you enjoy.

Then, begin with Level 1—whatever aerobic endurance training you like. I will go into more detail about Level 1 aerobic training: science-proven cycling, science-proven treadmill training, and sports-activities RSB in Chapters 7, 8, and 10. If you haven't tried some PD aerobic programs outlined in this book, try them out. Experiencing different kinds of aerobic classes before deciding what to do is essential. I recommend taking the time to watch a class or two if you are unsure of what type of aerobic endurance training you want to try. Instructors love to have people come and watch a lesson. Just let them know ahead of time that you would like to observe the class. Halfway through, you may be ready to jump in and join in the fun.

Remember Mikey in the 1972 Life Cereal Ad—Try It, You Might Like It? Let's Start With Level 1

I often find that people who think they won't like boxing end up loving it, and the same goes for treadmill classes or cycling. The first goal is to perform aerobic endurance training three times a week—Level 1. This exercise can be treadmill training, cycling, elliptical, stair climbing, and swimming, to name a few. If you are limited on time and can only squeeze in a few workouts a week, your best bet is working with a personal trainer or exercise professional who works with PWPD and create a circuit workout (combining aerobic and resistance training that involves doing each set of exercises one after the other with little or no rest in between) or going to a RSB class that does a circuit workout.

Remember, at first, you may start Level 1 exercise workouts only one day a week and gradually work your way up to three days a week. The same goes for the duration. If you are a beginner, start with as much time as you can manage (even if it's 10 minutes) and slowly work up to exercise for 30—45 minutes. Likewise, you can start with intervals (short bursts of exercise followed by recoveries). So you could work for thirty seconds to a minute at 80% MHR and then take the same time off and recover. Even if the class is doing something else, always work at your own pace until you can keep up with the pace of the class. There is no reason to rush anything. Before you know it, the exercise will become easier as your aerobic base builds.

Mix and Match Levels 2, 3, and 4, Based on What Symptoms You Want to Work On

The subsequent three levels of your PD Exercise Cocktail Plan™ depend on your disease stage, goals, and any medical conditions. Talk with your physical therapist or exercise professional who works with PD to see how to mix and match the three levels to align with your goals. For example, my client Julie Aufden-kamp (age 62) has a rare neurological disease called posterior column ataxia with retinitis pigmentosa (PCARP)—a genetic condition that affects vision and the nervous system.

Approximately 1,000 people in the U.S. have PCARP. Julie was diagnosed at the age of eight with progressive loss of sight. By the time she was 14 years old, she had lost 90% of her vision and currently has only 2% remaining. She worked as a life vocational rehabilitation counselor for the Iowa Department for the Blind.

Julie's neurologist sent her to me to help her work on balance, coordination, proprioception (the sense of self movement), endurance, and strength. Her cocktail of choice is Redd's Wicked Apple Ale, to which she applied her Exercise Cocktail Plan™ slogan, "Gonna beat ya to the core!"

Julie was an athlete in her youth and looked forward to bringing movement back to her life. She couldn't wait to cycle, so we put her on a bike. Julie loved it, and thus found her Level 1 exercise. I also asked her how she would do following only verbal cues during a Total HealthWorks Total Parkinson's class, which would help with balance, coordination, and proprioception. "Let's find out," Julie quipped. Well, I have to say, that she can follow better than half the people that can see. We found her the perfect Level 2 class.

Julie shared, "Working in Kristine's neuro program has profoundly impacted my life physically and emotionally. I was boosting my balance, coordination and building strength. I also improved aerobically, especially with endurance. But the biggest part for me was how much my confidence grew."

Looking down the road, we will see if yoga (for her Level 3 exercise) and strength training will address the other areas Julie is interested in developing. It's important to realize that plans change as people go through different stages of life or if their health needs change and they need to adjust.

There Are Many PD-Specific Classes to Choose From for Level 2

NOTE: Most of these classes do have a monetary cost involved. You will need to check with Medicare or other insurer to see if the classes that interest you are covered. You will also need to go to the website or call the program to determine the costs involved. Some online classes are offered at no cost, but not all. Check with each program to find out more details.

Level 2 in the PD Exercise Cocktail Plan™ is PD-specific work—classes that work on the things that PD takes away—arm swing, walking with a normal gait, loss of voice, etc. PD-specific classes include brain work, memory, balance, multitasking, natural gait movement, voice amplification, and large-amplitude walking. You can find this kind of work in the following PD classes. Below are some resources (in alphabetical order).

- **American Parkinson's Disease Association** (APDA): The APDA calendar of virtual events is a list of all PD programs and classes available online, and you can participate no matter where you live. They have a variety of PD-specific classes. Go to apdaparkinson.org/upcoming-events.

- **Dance for PD** is an internationally acclaimed program that offers research-backed dance classes for people with Parkinson's disease online, in New York City, and in 28 countries worldwide through a network of partners and associates. Free classes are available on Zoom. Join NYC headquarters and certified teachers from around the world in these interactive group classes. Go to danceforparkinsons.org.

- **LSVT BIG Therapy** teaches PWPD to use their bodies more normally. It trains people in improved movements for any activity, whether "small-motor" tasks like buttoning a shirt, "large-motor" tasks like getting up from a sofa or chair, or simply maintaining balance while walking. Go to lsvtglobal.

- **LSVT LOUD® Therapy** is an effective speech treatment for people with PD and other neurological conditions. Go to lsvtglobal.com

- **Movement Revolution**, a Parkinson's Foundation-Accredited program, offers a Neuro-Intensive Virtual Training Center. You can access virtual exercise programs, one-on-one personal training, and Rock Steady Boxing. The organization also has live centers in Chicago and the surrounding area. Go to movement-revolution.com.

- **PARTE™** provides a creative, drama-based outlet for PWPD and their care partners. The theater work inspires this program's exercises to target symptoms of PD. Training is offered to physical therapists, occupational therapists, speech therapists, and other professionals. The headquarters is in Kansas City. Go to jointheparte.com

- **Parkinson's Foundation** has PD "Live every Friday exercise classes online." You can go to parkinson.org and search for exercise classes (classes are free).

- **PWR!Moves®** is a PD-specific exercise program that "works to improve neuroplasticity and slow the progression of PD." This is a Tucson-based facility that founded its system in physical therapy for PD. They focus on big movements and target four critical skills that the disease attacks: antigravity extension, weight shifting, axial mobility, and transitional movements. In addition, this program has trained Parkinson Wellness Recovery (PWR) professionals across the country, and you can find a directory on their website. Finally, they offer virtual PD classes with a wide range of PD-specific training. They also offer training for exercise professionals. Go to pwr4life.org.

- **SPEAK OUT!® & LOUD Crowd®** help PWPD regain and maintain their speaking abilities through education, individual speech therapy, daily home practice, group sessions, and regular reassessments. Go to parkinsonvoiceproject.org.

- **Total HealthWorks (THW) Total Parkinson's** Founders Jackie Russell and David Zid (who were also the founders of Delay the Disease™) provide a wide range of classes online. Total Parkinson's incorporates rounds of cardio followed by PD-specific work (memory, large-amplitude walking, balance, multitasking, etc.). Strength and core work are also part of the training. Go to totalhealthworks.com for more information on classes and training for exercise professionals.

- **Urban Poling (ACE-ACSM-Approved)** is an outdoor exercise class for PWPD that increases mobility and function for every age, ability, and fitness level. Also known as Nordic Walking, the class utilizes Activator Poles™ (urbanpoling.com/urban-poles-us) to encourage good posture and provide additional stability. They also offer training for exercise professionals. Go to urban-poling.com.

As you can see, there are many kinds of classes to choose from for PD-specific work. Explore all of these. Other classes and programs may be found in your local area.

Level 3: Progressive Resistance Training Can Come from Personal Training or Classes That Have Strength Training Built into Them

I will go into more detail about progressive strength training in Chapter 9. However, for safety reasons, PWPD who undertake this training should work one-on-one with a certified personal trainer (CPT) if possible—someone who has the experience and education to work with PWPD. If you cannot afford to work with a personal trainer, classes like Rock Steady Boxing, Total HealthWorks's Total Parkinson's, and PWR!Moves® have strength training incorporated into their live workouts or available on their websites. In addition, Rock Steady Boxing now offers one-on-one personalized training for people who need more assistance than can be accommodated in a class—this allows PD workout plans to incorporate more strength training.

Level 4: Flexibility, Balance, and Stretching

Exercise and daily stretching have been shown to reduce rigidity (Borrione et al. 135) for PWPD. It also helps your muscles and joints stay flexible, which makes getting through the day much more manageable. Level 4, which includes flexibility, balance, and stretching, has several options to choose from:

- Tai Chi improves a person's balance and ability to walk and move steadily, and thus is an effective therapy for PWPD. Tai Chi classes focus on posture, breathing techniques, mindfulness, and learning to concentrate on weight shift and balance. A 2019 article titled *Tai Chi Versus Routine Exercise in Patients with Early- or Mild-Stage Parkinson's Disease: A Retrospective Cohort Analysis* (Li et al. 1-7) describes the research. Five hundred PWPD were divided into two groups: the TC group received 80 minutes per day of Tai Chi three times per week for two months, and the control group, RE, received 90 minutes of routine exercise (treadmill and dance) three times per week for two months. The Tai Chi group saw a decrease in their daily dose of levodopa or equivalent treatment, and 9% were successful in withdrawing for levodopa or equivalent treatment. The incidence of falls within six months of treatment was reduced in both groups, but "Tai Chi decreased incidence of falls significantly more than routine exercise" (Li et al. 3-7).

- Yoga has proven to be a practical class for PWPD. It helps improve functional mobility, balance, and lower-limb strength. In addition, students' moods improve as well as their sleep quality. A 2018 research article titled *Functional Improvements in Parkinson's Disease Following a Randomized Trial of Yoga* (Van Puymbroeck et al. 2018) found that "functional improvements in motor function, balance, gait, and freezing of gait indicate that this yoga intervention was successful in reducing fall risk in individuals with PD" (Van Puymbroeck et al. 6). You can find a free (donations encouraged) Adaptive Online Yoga for MS, Parkinson's, and Disabilities class at yogamovesms.org (recommended for Stages 1 and 2 PWPD).

- Neuro-Pilates and Pilates are more great options for flexibility, stretching, and strength. Pilates has a positive impact on fitness, balance, and physical function. A 2019 review titled *Benefits of Pilates in Parkinson's Disease: A Systematic Review and Meta-Analysis* (Suárez-Iglesias et al. 2019) looked at how Pilates can be safely prescribed for people with mild-to-moderate PD. "Preliminary evidence indicates that its practice could have a positive impact on fitness, balance, and physical function. Its benefits on lower-body function appear to be superior to those of other conventional exercises" (Suárez-Iglesias et al. 1). The Neuro Studio offers a fourteen-day free trial for classes. Go to online.theneurostudio (recommended for Stages 1 and 2 PWPD).

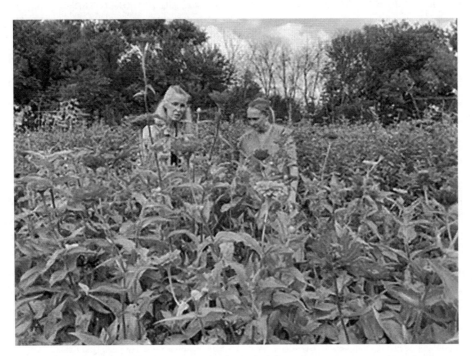

Level 5: Do what you love. Jane Collison, a PWPD, has extensive acreage where she grows vegetables and flowers. Jane and her husband, Bob, take the vegetables to local food banks. Jane and her PD friends also make flower arrangements to deliver to PWPD and retirement homes.

Level 5 Is Adding Things that You Love

The last part of the PD Exercise Cocktail Plan™ is Level 5—taking time to do things you love. Incorporating something that brings joy into your daily life is especially important. It can be anything—knitting, singing, golfing, painting, needlepoint, canoeing, hiking, bird watching, sightseeing, etc. Jane Collison (age 64), a retired business manager, LOVES to garden—that's a bit of an understatement (see Jane's story in Chapter 8). Jane has an extensive garden and grows flowers and vegetables to share with PWPD, retirement homes, and food banks. When Jane isn't working out, she is in the garden with her husband, Bob, or delivering her treasures to people in the community.

Industry Leaders Come Together to Create PD Exercise Recommendations for Exercise Professionals Who Work With PWPD

In 2020, the Parkinson's Foundation convened a meeting with a group of experts who identified a need to update PD exercise guidelines and build a competency framework for exercise professionals who work with PWPD. Attending were representatives from the American College of Sports Medicine (ACSM), the American Council on Exercise (ACE), the co-founders of Rock Steady Boxing, the co-founders of Total HealthWorks (then founders of Delay the Disease™), the Brian Grant Foundation, Dr. Jay Alberts, PhD, and others.

To achieve that end, committees were formed to develop professional competencies and exercise guidelines, explore partnerships with other stakeholders in the exercise and professional PD communities, and publish the resultant competencies and guidelines. Subsequent activities will address the feasibility of creating a Parkinson's Foundation Recognition Program to identify suitable exercise education programs (see Appendix A).

Lisa Hoffman, MA, director of Professional Education for the Parkinson's Foundation, explains that "The Parkinson's Foundation makes life better for people with Parkinson's disease (PD) by improving care and advancing research toward a cure. We know that medication is a vital component of treatment. We also know that exercise is just as essential and can even slow the progression of the disease. The Parkinson's Foundation encourages PWPD to participate in physical activity regularly and often; therefore, we must know what is good, what is valuable, what is a waste of time and money, and what is equitable. We know exercise is part of the treatment plan for people with Parkinson's. We say it, and now, we're putting our money and muscle behind the idea as we determined what it takes for an exercise professional to be competent to work with PWPD" (see Appendix B).

See Figure 3: Parkinson's Exercise Recommendations Chart.

Parkinson's Exercise Recommendations

Parkinson's is a progressive disease of the nervous system marked by tremor, stiffness, slow movement and balance problems.

Exercise and physical activity can improve many motor and non-motor Parkinson's symptoms:

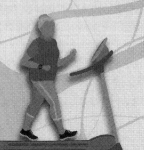

Aerobic Activity	Strength Training	Balance, Agility & Multitasking	Stretching
3 days/week for at least 30 mins per session of continuous or intermittent at moderate to vigorous intensity	2-3 non-consecutive days/week for at least 30 mins per session of 10-15 reps for major muscle groups; resistance, speed or power focus	2-3 days/week with daily integration if possible	>2-3 days/week with daily being most effective
TYPE: Continuous, rhythmic activities such as brisk walking, running, cycling, swimming, aerobics class	**TYPE:** Major muscle groups of upper/lower extremities such as using weight machines, resistance bands, light/moderate handheld weights or body weight	**TYPE:** Multi-directional stepping, weight shifting, dynamic balance activities, large movements, multitasking such as yoga, tai chi, dance, boxing	**TYPE:** Sustained stretching with deep breathing or dynamic stretching before exercise
CONSIDERATIONS: Safety concerns due to risks of freezing of gait, low blood pressure, blunted heart rate response. Supervision may be required.	**CONSIDERATIONS:** Muscle stiffness or postural instability may hinder full range of motion.	**CONSIDERATIONS:** Safety concerns with cognitive and balance problems. Hold on to something stable as needed. Supervision may be required.	**CONSIDERATIONS:** May require adaptations for flexed posture, osteoporosis and pain.

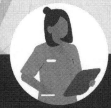

See a physical therapist specializing in Parkinson's for full functional evaluation and recommendations.

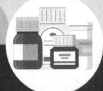

Safety first: Exercise during on periods, when taking medication. If not safe to exercise on your own, have someone with you.

It's important to **modify and progress** your exercise routine over time.

Participate in **150 minutes** of moderate-to-vigorous exercise per week.

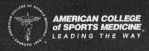
AMERICAN COLLEGE of SPORTS MEDICINE. LEADING THE WAY

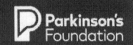
Parkinson's Foundation

Helpline: 800.473.4636/Parkinson.org

Figure 3: Parkinson's Exercise Recommendations Chart
Reprinted with permission from the Parkinson's Foundation 2023

As you go through the Parkinson's exercise recommendations for PD exercise, here are some additional things to think about.

Aerobic Section: The main exercise set should be flanked by a five-to-ten-minute warm-up and cooldown, particularly given the prevalence of autonomic dysfunction (Klanbut qtd. by Alberts and Rosenfeldt 2020 s24).

Strength Training: Power focus is not referring to "powerlifting" but to power training that involves performing concentric actions (the portion of the exercise when you are actually lifting the weight) explosively up to maximal exertion. Muscle power has been shown to promote improvement in a person's ability to perform daily activities. And the ability to generate extra power has an impact on things we don't necessarily think about—such as lifting a heavy bag of groceries to the counter.

Additional Key Considerations: When starting any exercise program, PWPD should consult with their neurologist or family physician to ensure they can safely engage in and complete any exercise program—many programs require a physician's release or a liability waiver to participate. It's best to consult with a PD physical therapist or experienced exercise professional who works with PWPD to guide you. Formal exercise guidance can help with the accountability and motivation necessary to overcome a lack of exercise self-efficacy (the confidence in one's ability to succeed) and depression that often accompanies PD.

If you require extra assistance throughout a class or feel that you are at high risk of falling, please ensure you have someone in your family or a friend to stay with you during the course of exercise. In RSB, they call this person your "cornerman." Some facilities may have volunteers to help you; however, this is not the normal procedure. While PD exercise classes are designed to work with people in different stages of PD, the Parkinson's Foundation recommends PWPD start exercising with a physical therapist before moving to organized group exercise programs.

CHAPTER 6

Exercise and Tools to Help Manage Your Workouts

"Chris[topher] Reeve wisely parsed the difference between optimism and hope. Unlike optimism, he said, "Hope is the product of knowledge and the projection of where the knowledge can take us."

- Michael J. Fox

Living as a PD Care Partner Is One of the Hardest Jobs in the World

My client Linda (age 79) was Leonard's primary care partner for over twenty years. Leonard, her husband, was diagnosed with PD in 2000, before most of the research on the benefit of PD exercise was published. He experienced a stiff shuffling gait, rigidity, and tremor. He did, however, hop on an Airdyne bike three times a week (those bikes with the arms you push back and forth while you ride) and felt symptom relief. Linda said, "Leonard liked his Airdyne bike so much he had two, one at home and one he kept in the travel trailer to take with us wherever we went. Later, he moved to a NuStep Recumbent cross-trainer, but I just remember that exercise helped him a great deal, and it was before we even knew how much exercise helped reduce PD symptoms."

When Linda Was Also Diagnosed With Parkinson's, They Had Challenging Decisions to Make

Linda felt at home in the care partner role because, she said, this was in her makeup and something she naturally embraced. It was not easy for them because Leonard had other illnesses besides PD, and the couple faced several surgeries together. However, the most difficult trial they endured as a married couple was when Linda was diagnosed with PD as well. "I really couldn't believe it that I had Parkinson's," said Linda. "Leonard knew what I was in for, having PD, and he didn't want me to go through it." It was a tough time for them. Linda didn't want to burden Leonard with her PD, and Leonard didn't want to burden her anymore, especially since she was also having PD symptoms. You might think, how could they have both gotten PD? The one common denominator was that they both either worked on or lived on farms.

Linda and Leonard were in a tough situation, faced with hard decisions based on her diagnosis. Leonard had been in the hospital to have a pacemaker installed, and he had gone to a rehabilitation nursing home to recover. Leonard was a big man whom Linda could not lift on her own. He couldn't walk alone and was susceptible to falling since he was in the later stages of PD. They had been wrestling with what to do to

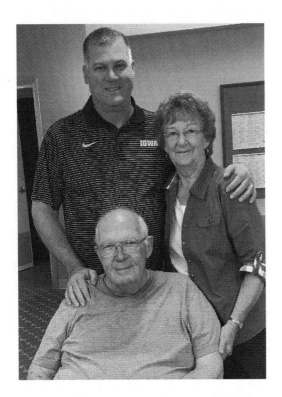

Linda O'Hair, with her husband, Leonard, and son, Greg. Linda cared for Leonard, who had PD, for twenty years. When Leonard had complications and was moved into a retirement home for recovery, the family found out Linda also had PD.

keep him safe, but with Linda's diagnosis, they had their answer. Leonard would have to stay in the nursing home. Unfortunately, PWPD and their care partners must make these difficult decisions throughout their lives, decisions that impact the entire family. Fortunately, Linda and Leonard had support from their family, friends, and the PD community.

Linda Recognized Her PD Symptoms Right Away

When I interviewed Linda, I asked if she knew she had PD immediately. Most people don't recognize or understand the symptoms of PD, especially since they often happen gradually, and the early symptoms are overlooked. However, Linda had been front row to her husband's disease progression, so I felt she would know when symptoms appeared. Linda answered, "Yes, I knew. I noticed my symptoms when trying to curl my hair or do my makeup. . I'd slightly shake. Then I fell for no reason. I would fall into the grass or the leaves all the time while I was out doing simple chores. But the main giveaway was my writing. December 2017, I couldn't write or even sign our Christmas cards, let alone write a note. So, I took my journal and wrote in it to show the neurologist at my March appointment. I just knew it then. I truly had PD."

Linda Misses Her Sweetheart— She Seldom Missed a Day Visiting Him during COVID-19

For three years, from the time Leonard went to stay full time in the nursing home, Linda visited Leonard, seldom missing a day. Even when the COVID-19 pandemic came and she wasn't allowed to enter the building, she would go to his window. They would talk on the phone and spend time with each other. Linda was always leaving cycle class to go see her "sweetheart," and we were always moved by her devotion and love for Leonard. He passed on Monday, January 25, 2021, in the arms of his sweetheart, Linda.

For Someone Who Wasn't a Big Exercise Enthusiast in Her Youth, She Is Crushing It Now

Linda joined my neuro-cycling program shortly after she was diagnosed in 2018. She told me her favorite drink was a margarita. Her PD Exercise Cocktail Plan™ is called the "Margarita Crush It." Like so many women I have met, Linda found that boxing is much more fun than she thought it would be. She said, "I like Rock Steady Boxing and all the aerobic exercises that go along with that. It isn't that we box all the time. I like the camaraderie we have, as well as the discipline and consistency the class provides. The coach is wonderful—that makes a big difference."

Cycling Isn't Her Favorite, But She Loves What It Does for Her Brain and Symptoms

Even though Linda started cycling as her first PD exercise choice, she has mixed feelings about it. While it may not be her favorite exercise, she gets excellent results for her PD symptoms from it. She has this to say about cycling: "What's the hardest for me? It's cycling. But I know it makes a big difference. And I think it makes a difference for many people because we have the same people coming back all the time."

Battling PD Takes Perseverance and the Ability to Not Back Down

If there was one word to describe Linda, it would be perseverance. She doesn't back down from PD, and she takes life and all its challenges in stride. She is also a warm and caring person to everyone around her. As her coach, I'm grateful she has children who actively support her as caretakers, since she spent much of her life as a caretaker herself.

Aren't Exercise and Physical Activity the Same? No! I'm Sorry to Say They Are Not

Let's discuss the difference between exercise and physical activity. When I talk to people around the country, many feel that "gardening" and "walking the dog" are exercise workouts. Don't get me wrong, I walk my dogs two miles daily and I love to garden. But I consider this as physical activity, not my daily exercise.

Dog walking and gardening belong in Level 5 of the PD Exercise Cocktail Plan™, the "Do what you love" category. Dr. Alberts says, "Too often, people with Parkinson's are told that exercise is good without being given any sense of what type or how much exercise." He further explains, "Patients are given advice like, 'If you like to garden, then you should garden.' Now gardening is a nice physical activity, but it's not exercising at a high enough intensity level to be neuroprotective. If we want to treat exercise as medicine for this disease, we need to provide patients with an actual prescription that specifies frequency, duration, intensity, and heart rate."

Exercise and physical activity are two different things. "Physical activity is defined as any bodily movement produced by skeletal muscles that results in energy expenditure . . . Exercise is a subset of physical activity that is planned, structured, and repetitive and has as a final or an intermediate objective—the improvement or maintenance of physical fitness" (Caspersen et al. 126).

Chapter 6

Physical activity and exercise play a role in the management and quality of life of PWPD. Exercise is a broad term that includes aerobic exercise, strength training, flexibility training, and others. This distinction is important because, for too long, PWPD have been hearing from different sources that physical activity is exercise. If your goal is to hopefully slow disease progression and reduce symptoms, physical activity alone will not help you achieve that. Exercise will!

Measuring With Heart Rate or Perceived Exertion Scale

Your active heart rate is a measurement of your heart activity, in heartbeats per minute, during exercise. People can use it to optimize their workouts by ensuring that their heart rate stays within the ideal range—for our purposes, it is to make sure we hit the target of 80% of maximum heart rate (MHR). MHR is as fast as your heart can beat.

One attempt to determine MHR was Haskell's equation (subtracting the subject's age from 220), which was designed in the 1970s. However, that equation was based on a group that likely included "subjects with cardiovascular disease who smoked and/or were taking cardiac medications. Each of these conditions influences [MHR] independent of age" (Tanaka et al. 155). Haskell's equation was not intended to become the standard metric for finding a healthy person's MHR, but somehow, it did.

The Tanaka equation (208 minus 0.7 times age) is the formula currently recommended by the National Academy of Sports Medicine (NASM). This equation is not perfect, but it works better than the Haskell equation to get you close to your correct 80% MHR number. So, using the Tanaka method, see Figure 4 for the formula for a person who is 60 years old.

Tanaka Formula

208 - (0.7 x age) = HRmax
80 % of HR max

Example for a 60-year-old:

208 - (0.7 x age) = HRmax
208 - (0.7 x 60) = HRmax
208 - (42) = 166
80% of 166 = 132

Note: If you need to start at a lower % of HRmax, just put in the number that works for you.

Figure 4: The Tanaka heart rate formula example.

Target Heart Rate

It's essential to understand your personal target heart rate range while you work out. You want to work out hard enough to reach your target, but don't overdo it. Your target heart rate is how fast you want your your working intensity. Your target heart rate will depend on your current fitness level and age, which means it will change as your cardiovascular endurance increases or as you age. Your target heart rate is how fast you want your heart rate to beat while exercising. The heart rate reflected on the treadmill monitor when you grab the heart rate handle sensor or look at the heart rate application on the watch you wear will indicate your exercise.

Determining Heart Rate by Perceived Exertion

There are two ways to determine if you are working at the 80% MHR level. One is by heart rate, and the other is by perceived exertion. A heart-rate zone is a specific heart-rate range, measured in beats per minute and calculated as a percentage of your estimated MHR, used to monitor training intensity during exercise

If measuring your heart rate using the Tanaka equation won't work because your medications will affect its outcome, we have a different measurement tool—the Rate of Perceived Exertion Scale (RPE). Of course, this method is subjective, so you must be honest about how hard you're working. The RPE scale ranges from one to ten, with ten being the highest difficulty level (see Figure 5). Thus, 80%–85% of maximum heart rate would put you between numbers 4-6 (Moderate Activity) and 7–8 (Moderate to Vigorous), as shown in Figure 5.

Work Slowly to Build Up Your Cardio Base Over Time

As a beginner or someone just getting back to exercise, you will quickly hit your 80% MHR (you will feel breathless and winded) because you don't have a solid aerobic base built. Because of that, it's essential to be careful and not overdo your aerobic effort initially. Pay attention to what your body tells you when you are working at higher efforts. If you have any medical concerns or conditions, you should consult your physician about the suitable heart rate range you should be working within for your situation. Likewise, if you have heart conditions, consult your physician on what ranges you should stay within for safety and what to avoid.

The key to building your aerobic base will depend upon your consistency in workouts. It will take six to eight weeks to build up your cardio base. After that, it will get easier to hit higher levels of intensity. Then you can extend the duration that your heart rate is elevated. Start at an aerobic level you are comfortable with, no matter what the heart rate number, and have fun. Enjoy the process.

Rate of Perceived Exertion (RPE) Scale

1	**VERY LIGHT** It doesn't feel like exercise.
2-3	**LIGHT** You can do this all day. Walk, talk, and breathe.
4-5	**MODERATE** You notice your breathing, but you can hold a conversation.
6-7	**DIFFICULT** You can talk, but your breathing is elevated.
8-9	**VERY DIFFICULT** You can say a few words. It's hard to breathe.
10	**MAX EFFORT** You're out of breath and can't talk.

Figure 5: The RPE Rate of Perceived Exertion Scale can help you "feel" where to work from when you are doing aerobic training. Use this scale if the heart-rate method won't work for you.

CHAPTER 7

Parkinson's Science-Proven Exercise: PD Cycling

"Basketball gave me a life;
Parkinson's taught me how to live it."

– Brian Grant, author and former NBA star

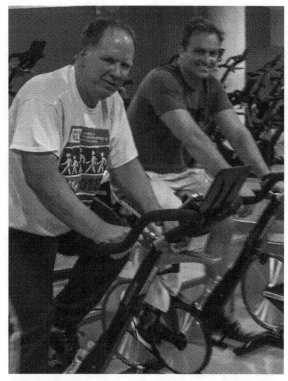

Jim Best (left) and his son, Greg, ride together in a Neuro-cycle class. It is important for family members to work out with PWPD, who are so happy to have the support of loved ones as they exercise.

Staying Positive Is a Must in the Daily Battle with PD

Life had already been difficult for Jim Best. His dad died and then his brother died. Upon his brother's death, the aftermath of unresolved issues of the family construction business was dumped into Jim's lap to take care of, along with the other family problems. Just when he had climbed out of the abyss and thought life would improve, he was told he had PD. He was in his 50s. Jim said, "You just have to stay positive, and if you do, you've already won half the day's battle with Parkinson's." Jim loves to be silly, and he spreads positivity wherever he goes. Jim was one of the first PWPD I had the privilege to work with, and he makes me laugh and smile daily. Whenever I play Charlie Daniels' song "The Devil Goes Down to Georgia" in class, I smile and think of Jim because it is his favorite song to cycle to—he loves to get the whole class to sing.

When I interviewed him, we reminisced about the good old days, with our "starter" PD group. We had fun classes, parties, social events, and even a Live-to-Tri Triathlon. That's right, my Neuro Wellness class designed a triathlon for everyone who wanted to try a triathlon but needed it designed especially for them. They planned the event with a few stipulations:

1. They didn't want to walk around in wet bathing suits for the event. Who can blame them! So, they made the swim portion last for ten minutes at the end of the triathlon, and they could march, walk, or swim in the pool.

2. They agreed they could handle a twenty-minute walk/jog around the track using whatever device they needed (canes, walkers, etc.). However, they also had the option to use the treadmill.

3. They said they could "kick ass" on the bike and wanted to cycle for forty-five minutes. However, I told them to think about others who hadn't been cycling as much as they had, so they relented and agreed to thirty minutes.

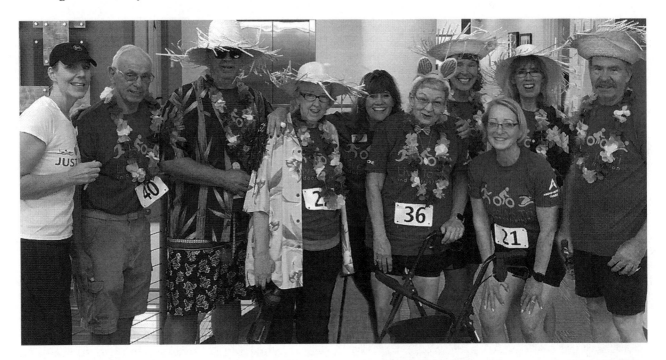

Some of the Live to Tri PD crew: (left to right) Chantelle Smith, Ray Paul Pietig, Jim Best, Sandy Trent, Kristine Meldrum, Mary Fran Pietig, Cristina Bucksbaum, Jen Voorhees, Jane Collison and Pat Ferring. It was Jim Best's idea for them to dress up for our group triathlon. The group designed the Live to Tri triathlon—a twenty-minute walk/run on the track, a thirty-minute cycle ride, and a ten-minute walk/swim in the pool. Everyone had a great time during the event. A big celebration was held afterward, complete with tri-goodie bags and fun prizes.

The event was open to PWPD, to members of Above + Beyond Cancer (a local cancer-survivor group), and to anyone who ever wanted to do a triathlon but felt intimidated. It was a memorable day; competitors completed the event with big smiles on their faces.

Jim had started working with me at a hospital health workout center where I taught for a decade, but when I left to build a full-scale neuro program elsewhere, he stayed behind because the health center was across the street from his house. It is one of the hardest things about the PD community; you form such strong bonds, and it is difficult when you spend every day together and then changes occur.

Jim Exercises Hard Every Day to Feel Like He Doesn't Have PD

Jim's favorite form of PD exercise is cycling. He came to all the cycling classes I taught—not just my PD cycle classes. He explained, "Cycling has always been the class I like the best, and what I felt I got the most

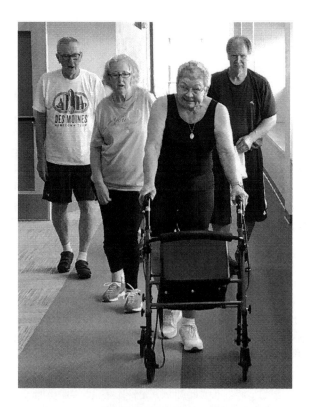

Pictured left to right: Bill Brown, Sandy Trent, Mary Fran Pietig, and Jim Best training on the track for the "walk/run" of the "Live to Tri" event. Others in the group used the treadmill for their training.

results for my symptoms from."

But he also likes boxing, aqua classes, and many others. He likes to keep moving, and there is a good reason for that. "Exercise is critical for me," explained Jim. "Because when I go to classes early in the day, it sets me up for two important hours later in the evening, two hours when I feel somewhat normal. My symptoms are subdued enough that I can go to dinner with my wife and not shake all over the place and I can speak without stuttering. Those two precious hours a day are what I want the most. And that's what exercise gives to me. A couple of hours where I don't feel like I have Parkinson's."

Helping Others With PD and Giving to the Community Is Important to Jim

Jim hopes that everyone with PD will find a way to let exercise help them with their PD journey. He has embraced movement for PD since he was diagnosed and wants others to know how important it is to stay healthy. Jim explains, "I have seen my friends with PD make a choice not to exercise and watched them deteriorate at a rapid pace. So I give anyone and everyone information about exercise because I don't want that to happen to them." Jim has a big heart and cares about his PD friends, his family, and those newly diagnosed and coming to the community. As one of the biggest supporters of the PD local community, Jim has made tremendous contributions to promote exercise in his community—including providing a financial donation for an entire boxing facility.

Find Your People and Let Them Support You

There is a beauty to PD exercise programs and classes—they provide a community of support to participants. Programs help people who aren't naturally motivated to exercise. PWPD quickly find that they want to go to classes because they are fun and they get to see their friends there. "It is important to note that short-term exercise is not the panacea to treating PWPD; improvements in motor symptoms following short-term exercise dissipate after four weeks of inactivity, indicating that the exercise, similar to antiparkinsonian medication, must be integrated into a PWPDs routine to achieve consistent benefits" (Alberts and Rosenfeldt S23). Exercise programs are a long-term solution for PWPD, and, as we know, PD is here for the long haul. For the PWPD, exercise must become a new way of life to keep PD in check.

Your Exercise Coach or Professional Sees Your Changes Before You Do

Another benefit to having an exercise professional who works with PWPD in your corner is that we see our people daily and sometimes twice a day. Because of our training and the fact that we are with them so much, we notice things about them that they may not notice. For instance, remember Bill, who had difficulty gaining back ground after COVID? Not long after COVID, he went in for a routine battery change on his DBS unit. It was a simple surgical procedure that had him out of the class for a few days, and then he was back. Shortly after this, I noticed Bill's balance was off, and he was not cycling at his regular cadence (revolutions per minute). I mentioned it to him. He said, "Now that you say that, I haven't felt quite 100%. But I just got the COVID vaccine, so I thought that was why I felt this way."

Another week went by, and Bill was not doing any better. I told him to call his neurologist and ask if it could be the new battery. The neurologist told him, "It can't be the battery. They hardly ever go bad. One in one hundred goes wrong. It's not the battery." So, we scratched our heads. Another week and a half went by, and Bill's exercise performance got even worse. I told him, "Call your neurologist and tell her I told you that you must be seen right now because something is wrong." Long story short, it was the battery. Bill was the one in one hundred!

As part of your PD care team, coaches have different roles and perspectives. We are here to support you on your daily journey with PD. And we ensure that you get the right resources and information for you to make informed decisions to stay healthy.

Let's Talk about Exercises You Can Choose to Help Manage Your PD Symptoms

In the next four chapters, I will go through three science-proven exercise endurance programs: cycling, treadmill, and progressive strength training. I will also discuss one sports-activities exercise program (boxing) to help you decide which aerobic programs you may want to try for your PD Exercise Cocktail Plan™. There are many more sports-activities exercise classes to choose from: dance, cardio aqua, Total HealthWorks' Total Parkinson's classes, and more. But I would need to write a second book to cover everything in this category.

The Difference Between Science-Proven Exercise and Sports Activities Exercise

The difference between a science-proven exercise and a sports-activities exercise is . . . a lot of research. Science-proven exercises like treadmill training for PD, cycling for PD, and progressive strength training for PD have more than twenty years of research behind them. What you have read in this book regarding research by Professor Corcos, Dr. Alberts, and Professor Bloem is the tip of the iceberg. There are a host of other scientists researching these areas, only a few of whom I have listed. Millions upon millions of dollars have been spent in research to prove the efficacy of these exercises.

Research in science-proven exercise has determined each program's optimum frequency, time, intensity, and type. So, that is the biggest difference between science-proven exercise and sports activities exercise (Corcos). Sports-activities exercises do have supporting research, depending on the individual program, but not nearly as much as the science-proven exercises. The sport-activities exercises also don't have clearly defined parameters of frequency, duration, intensity, and type determined through a large body of scientific research.

That is not to say the sports-activities exercise programs are not effective. They are highly effective for PWPD. While you will read in Chapter 10 about one—Rock Steady Boxing—there are many exceptional sports-activities exercise programs listed in this book as well. Even though they don't have as extensive research behind them as science-proven exercise programs, these programs can take the science-proven exercise information and build it into their program methodology.

The following three chapters will break down these exercise programs, discuss some history and science, detail the methodology of the training, and explain what a workout would entail.

PD Cycling or Neuro-Cycling Classes

Chapters 1 and 2 outlined extensive research regarding the benefits of cycling for PWPD. Over the years, Dr. Alberts implemented a nonprofit cycling program across the United States called "Pedaling for Parkinson's"™ (PFP). During COVID-19, many PFP sites closed, though you can still find online classes at pedalingforparkinsons.org. You can also find online cycling classes at the NCCA-ACE Approved Parkinson's Cycling Coach website: parkinsonscyclingcoach.com. There are also many neuro-cycling classes or PD cycling classes offered at different wellness centers, gyms, or YMCAs. Check with your local Parkinson's organizations for listings of exercise classes in your area.

What to Expect When You Go for Your Cycle Assessment

The rider is set up on an indoor bike with Bluetooth wireless technology that allows the rider to track the workouts—power, cadence, speed, heart rate, and more. A baseline metric assessment (a first measurement of where you started with cadence, power, and time, to track progress going forward) is administered. Riders are encouraged to start with a revolutions-per-minute (RPM) rate at which they are comfortable. They are then coached to gradually increase over time to ride at a pedaling rate that is faster than they would choose on their own. The goal is to ultimately get them cycling at a target cadence of 80 RPM. Now, before you think to yourself, "I can't do that," I want to assure you that this all happens in stages. No one hops on a bike in class and rides 80 RPM their first day—unless they have been biking their whole life. So don't jump to another chapter yet, and I will walk you through the process step by step below.

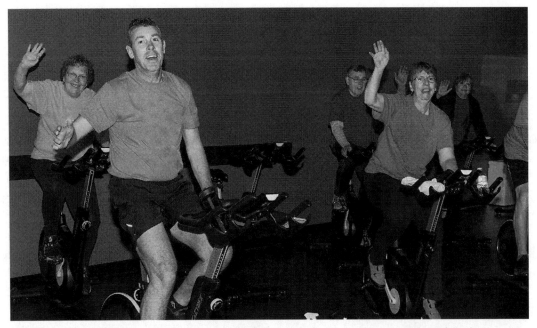

Neuro-cycling classes are fun. Look at the smiles on these faces. Pictured left to right in the back row: Kay Arvidson, Mike Hawkins, and Kim Robey. Front row left, to right: Joe Hingl and Carol Harvey. Most of these people didn't think they would like cycling before they decided to try it, but they quickly found out it is fun and does great things for their PD symptoms.

Photo by Laraine Davis

Proper Bike Setup Is Essential to Prevent Injuries to Your Back and Knees

Proper bike fitting is essential. The correct bike settings help prevent injuries, increase efficiency, provide comfort, and improve performance. With PWPD, it is crucial to have the knees aligned correctly and the seat and handlebars in the proper position. Every bike is different, and you must be refitted for each new type of bike you ride on. Settings don't transfer over to different types of bikes—a Peloton setting does not work for a Kaiser bike or a Schwinn and so forth.

What Happens When You Go to Your First Class?

First, group cycle PD classes are fun and I like to have interactive games between the rows of cyclists. My group comes up with goofy team names, like "Sloths" vs. "Lightning Bolts," for interval work (short bursts of work followed by short segments of rest). When new PWPD join the 45-minute class, they ride at their own pace for the time they want to participate, building up their aerobic capacity. I tell people, "If you can make it ten minutes on your first ride, you are doing great." And most people stop primarily because of cycle seat discomfort, not the aerobic part. I keep extra bike gel seats, so people don't have to leave due to seat discomfort.

The first time you go into a cycle class, and you decide it feels too overwhelming, split up your work into "bite-size" work sections. Maybe your goal is to make it for ten minutes. Great! Like any other class, you must build up your aerobic base, which means you will feel breathless quickly if you haven't been working out. You will work out in "on" and "off" patterns, regardless of what the class may be doing. "On" means working at a pace that makes you feel breathless. "Off" is your recovery time. So you would work "on" for one minute at your target RPM, which should put you at the right MHR, and then "off" for one minute for your ten minutes or however long you ride. You will also not work at too high of a cadence since you are just starting, but rather at an RPM just enough to feel like you are working. You will soon understand what you are doing, and it gets easier each time you ride the bike.

Cycling Training Case Studies
Cidney and Pat Donahoo (Las Vegas, Nevada)

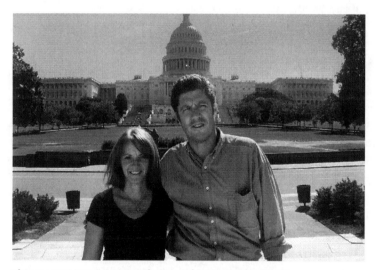

Cidney and Pat Donahoo in Washinton, DC, in 2006.

You Never Know When Life Is Going to Throw You a Curve Ball

During a family celebration trip to Washington, DC, in 2006, with their oldest son, who had just graduated from high school, a small observation would forever change the entire trajectory of Cidney and Pat Donahoo's lives. "She was just walking kind of funny," explained Pat. "Her right arm wasn't swinging, and she looked stiff." Cidney was young—only 44 years old. Cidney spent the next three years going to doctors, trying to figure out what was going on. Her only other symptom was a twitch in her pinkie.

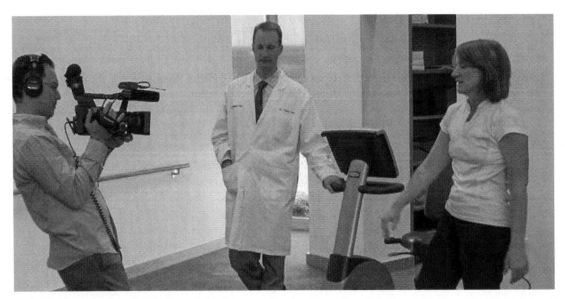

Dr. Jay Alberts with Cidney Donahoo, who was part of Dr. Albert's follow-on "Forced vs. Voluntary" cycle studies for PWPD, in Las Vegas, Nevada.

Cidney Sought Out Dr. Jay Alberts and His PD Cycling Clinical Trial

Cidney explained, "I finally started looking it up online, and I mentioned Parkinson's to my neurologist. And he goes, 'No, no, no, you don't have Parkinson's, but you have Parkinsonism.' And I'm like, 'What does that even mean?' So, I went online and looked up the difference. I said to him, 'I don't think so, I think I have Parkinson's.' But he never diagnosed me."

Frustrated, and rightly so, Cidney went to the Cleveland Clinic in Las Vegas, Nevada, where she lived. Cidney said, "I had heard about all the research at the Cleveland Clinic, specifically by Dr. Jay Alberts, the *Forced, Not Voluntary, Exercise Improves Motor Function in Parkinson's Disease* clinical trial. So, I finally got diagnosed with Parkinson's disease by a doctor at the Cleveland Clinic. I hadn't ridden a bike since I was a child, but I wanted to be part of a study and see if it helped my PD," continued Cidney. "I was fortunate to participate in one of Dr. Jay Albert's cycle studies from 2010 to 2011."

You Don't Have a Bike, and Where the Hell's Iowa?

During the study, Cidney became friends with the research assistant, Kathy Nagel, who was going to participate that summer in RAGBRAI—the Register's Annual Great Bicycle Ride Across Iowa. That year, 8,500 people registered to participate in RAGBRAI, an annual seven-day, 500-mile bicycle ride across the state. Having participated in Dr. Albert's bike study and feeling great, Cidney wanted to go too.

She went home to Pat and proudly proclaimed she would ride a bike across Iowa. Pat replied, "You don't have a bike, and where the hell's Iowa? What do you mean you're going to ride 500 miles across Iowa?"

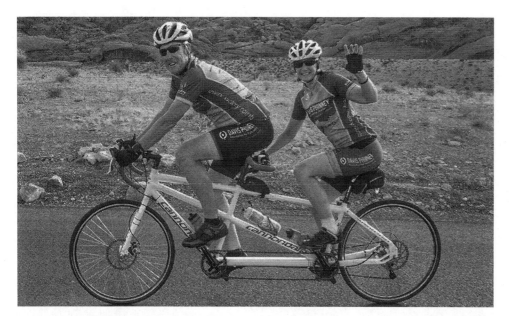

Neither Pat nor Cidney rode bikes before Cidney was diagnosed with PD, but they both became avid cyclists to keep her symptoms under control. They have participated in many PD cycling events over the years.

But Pat bought her a bike, and Cidney rode 500 miles across Iowa. Pat became part of the PD care support team for RAGBRAI, and he even got on a bike and rode for a couple of days. After that experience, their lives changed.

Cycling Became an Integral Part of Their Everyday Lives— Something They Did Together

Cidney and Pat became avid bike riders. And for more than ten years this exercise kept Cidney's symptoms (which were mostly dyskinesia and rigidity) under control. When I asked Cidney how exercise improved her life, she said, "It became an integral part of our everyday life. Something we did together. And we both got into shape quickly and maintained that for a long, long time. The exercise worked so well for both motor and non-motor symptoms. I felt good, you know. I felt really good."

Earliest Ambassadors for the Davis Phinney Foundation for Parkinson's

Cidney and Pat continued riding their tandem bike all over the country. They were so enthusiastic about helping PWPD that they became involved with the Davis Phinney Foundation for Parkinson's. In fact, they were two of the earliest Davis Phinney Foundation Ambassadors—providing education and resources about PD to people in Nevada. In addition, they founded Parkinson's Place Las Vegas, a nonprofit organization that helps people with, and affected by, PD discover new possibilities and transform their lives.

Chapter 7

Finally, they hold a large yearly PD movement conference to present the latest information and exercises to help PWPD in their community understand the importance of exercise.

Words of Advice from Someone Who's Had PD for Seventeen Years

I asked Cidney if she were to talk to somebody who is newly diagnosed with PD what advice she would give that person about exercise. She answered, "Do it. Every day, if you can, and mix it up—cardio, strength, flexibility, brain training, all of it."

Cidney recently hurt her back and hasn't been able to exercise, and dyskinesia has reared its ugly head. The combination has kept her from her daily exercise. Cidney said, "I got really depressed and felt lots of anxiety when I hurt my back and couldn't work out. I stopped exercising, which is not like me, and my symptoms got out of control. So, I know I need to get back to exercising to feel better and in control of my PD."

> *Do It [exercise]. Every day, if you can, and mix it up—cardio, strength, flexibility, brain training, all of it.*
>
> **- Cidney Donahoo, PWPD**

PD changes the course of people's lives. It also teaches life lessons that are often surprising. I asked Cidney what she learned about herself from having PD. She answered, "Perseverance. I gained courage and a strong sense of perseverance. And our lives took paths they wouldn't have taken. I wouldn't have become a bike enthusiast for one—Pat wouldn't have either, as hard as it is to believe now. We wouldn't have become Ambassadors or started our Parkinson's nonprofit. When I think of all the amazing connections and thousands of people we've helped, it is a wonderful life."

PD Wants Me to Give Up, But I'm Not Going to Let It Win. We've Had This Battle Before. I Always Come Away the Victor

Having been diagnosed as a young-onset person, Cidney has had PD for a very long time. Throughout the years, things have gotten tough at various points. Cidney had to make hard decisions and break through the mental blocks PD threw her way.

She says, "I feel like right now I'm kind of in the middle of a rough patch, where PD wants me to give up, but I'm not going to let it win. We've had this battle before. I always come away the victor. It doesn't mean it's not a struggle when I'm in the middle of it. We each control our fight with PD. Arming ourselves with support and knowledge is the only way to help us come out on top. I just want you to know that everyone struggles, and it's okay. Just fight and win."

Cycling Training Case Studies
John Tomeny (Hanover, New Hampshire)

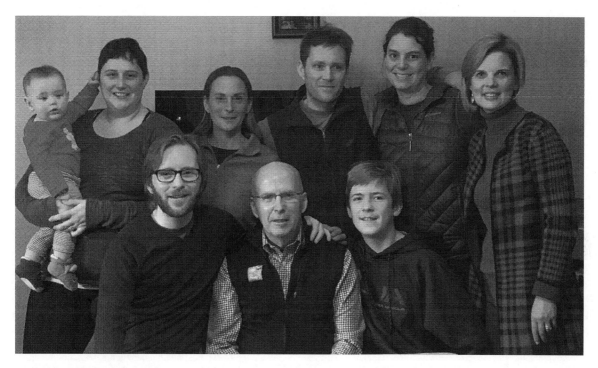

John Tomeny and his family.

When the Doctor Told Him He Had PD, He Thought the Absolute Worst

"My heart stopped. I didn't know a thing about Parkinson's. I didn't know if it was a death sentence. I didn't know how much longer I had to live. I had three children. Two of them were in high school, one was married and living in Maine. I hadn't had the opportunity to get to know her husband very well yet. My grandchildren had not been born yet. I always imagined holding them. My younger sons were not married yet. And I wanted to be there for their weddings," said John. All these thoughts rushed through his head after his doctor had told him in 2014 that he had PD.

Speechless and Unable to Say the Diagnosis, He Handed His Wife the Paper

His wife was sitting in the lobby waiting for him to tell her about the appointment. John said, "I was working as hard as I could to not cry. Finally, I walked up to her. And I couldn't speak. I was holding the discharge papers with the diagnosis written on them. I opened my mouth, and nothing came out. Just stood there with my mouth wide open. So, finally, I pointed to the diagnosis on the paper. She looked at me and said, 'You've got Parkinson's disease?' I said, 'Yeah, it says so there.'" John kept a stone face because he didn't want her to worry, but he was scared out of his mind. He sat down on the bench next to her. He said, "I'm sorry." It was a difficult situation. He knew that it would change their lives and their family. At the time of diagnosis, John was 63 years old.

The Journey That Led Him to This Point in Time

How did John get here? A few isolated incidents got him wondering what was going on with his body and mind. He and his wife were on Cape Cod, Massachusetts, jumping between stones on the jetties that cut the crosscurrents to prevent ocean riptides. As she leaped from boulder to boulder, John was trying to keep up with her. And it wasn't fatigue slowing him down. It was FEAR. John explained, "I suddenly had this irrational fear in my head as I was ready to leap to the next boulder. My brain was telling me, 'DON'T DO IT! You're not going to make it.' And I was like, wow, where did that thought come from anyway? But I froze and ended up crawling on my knees over the rocks to catch up with my wife."

While Teaching a Salsa Class, Things Didn't Happen Quite the Way They Should

They came back from vacation and got into their everyday routines. Things were going on as usual, and John forgot about his moment of fear.

Today John is 71, a retired IT Asset Management (ITAM) subject-matter expert, and an international ITAM standards author. During his career, he traveled and taught thousands of people worldwide how to use ITAM practices in their companies.

John thought the incident on the rocks was a thing of the past until two months after the Cape Cod vacation. John was teaching a salsa dance lesson, and he said to the class loudly, "Do what I do." His mind said, "Feet, dance," as he had done thousands of times, but his feet did nothing. His feet were stuck to the floor. Everybody was lined up in rows behind him, staring blankly. And some wise guy in the back row yells, "Do what I do. Uh-huh!" That pissed John off, so he stepped back with his right foot and started salsa dancing like nobody's business. However, the incident frightened John. He knew something was wrong, so he scheduled an exam with his neurologist, who happened to work with Dr. Jay Alberts on the *Forced versus Voluntary CYCLE* trial. She knew John liked to cycle, and she let him know about the amazing findings from the study.

Amazing Things Happen on the Annual Register's Great Bicycle Ride Across Iowa (RAGBRAI)

John met Jay Alberts years later at the Register's Annual Great Bicycle Ride Across Iowa (RAGBRAI). Cycling has always been the key to John keeping his symptoms under control. He is a cyclist through and

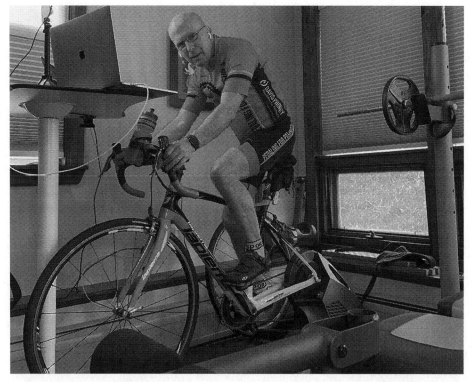

John Tomeny is a Pedaling for Parkinson's™ cycle instructor for PD students worldwide via Zoom.

through, riding 2,000 miles a year. When I asked John if he felt that exercise helped him slow the progression of his disease, he answered passionately, "Absolutely! Yes!" He then explained remorsefully that for a year and a half, he fell off the PD exercise wagon. John started fighting depression, his symptoms got worse, and he put on weight. He was miserable. Finally, things took a turn. "I found some inspiration and kept it for good," explained John. "I started working my ass off. And everything was so much better again—PD symptoms, depression, sleep, everything improved."

Giving Back to PWPD Is John's Way of Being Part of the Community

These days, John takes a multifaceted approach to his PD regimen. He has a personal trainer, Karlen, who strength trains him on a weekly basis. John also works with a nutritionist who gives him a meal plan and optimal food options for PD. John still cycles outdoors, but he also is a Pedaling for Parkinson's™ cycle instructor for PD students worldwide via Zoom (and he teaches salsa for PWPD). All of these things keep him on track. In addition, John enjoys giving back to the PD community. He volunteers for the Parkinson's Foundation and for a local group called the Upper Valley Programs for Parkinson's. He is also a Parkinson's Forum Ambassador to the U.S. Congress. He works hard to care for himself so that he can go out into the PD world and help others daily.

Chapter 7

The Four Pillars That Changed His Life Battling PD

I asked John what is a significant message that he shares from his experience when he speaks to PWPD. He said, "The first thing I tell them is PD is not a death sentence. It's a lifetime commitment. It's a challenge. One that will challenge you to excel. And it's a privilege. Because, as PWPD, we get to do things that other people can't do. We get to be miraculous people. That is, if we are willing. It is worth it to start being authentic and work harder than ever. And then, I tell them about the four pillars that changed my life. If you keep these four pillars in balance and manage them, you'll be successful in your journey with PD. It doesn't mean that you won't suffer along the way, but you'll be successful at giving yourself a life that you've never imagined having before. Those four pillars:

1) Sleep. Your body needs lots of rest and recovery.
2) Nutrition. The right fuel we put in our body helps reduce inflammation and gives us the energy for the third pillar.
3) Exercise. The most important of the pillars is exercise. Without exercise, we rapidly fall apart, and PD wins.
4) Hydration.

People often overlook the importance of hydrating the body, which is crucial for the average person and critical for PWPD (roughly 60% of our bodies are water)." John believes that when PWPD find balance with these four pillars, they will have what they need to succeed against PD.

The PD Journey Changed Him Into a Better Human Being

John explained that PD taught him more about himself and life than he would have learned if he hadn't gotten the disease. He recalled, "I didn't expect to find a community of people that were so positive, supportive, and well connected to each other. When I got PD, I entered a community of the most supportive people I've ever known, and that's why it's a privilege. I was often selfish and insensitive to others before PD. I've emerged as a different person since my diagnosis. I'm grateful for that, and I'm sure my friends and family are too."

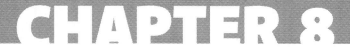

CHAPTER 8

Parkinson's Science-Proven Exercise: PD Treadmill

"Resolve never to quit, never to give up, no matter what the situation."

– Jack Nicklaus

Early-Onset PD Can Be Difficult to Adjustment When You Are First Wading through the PD Waters

Jane Collison wanted to walk out of the first PD exercise class she attended. It was shocking to her. She was only in her 50s, and the other people in the Delay the Disease™ class (aerobics class with PD work) were in their 60s to 80s and in various stages of the disease. It scared her to see where PD might ultimately take her. So, she left the class and didn't return; that is, until she was ready to face the music. "I felt like someone had gut-punched me. I didn't want to feel like that, and I felt guilty for feeling that way. Facing the reality of my disease was a tough pill for me to swallow. I had to process the truth staring me in the face and allow myself time to personally grieve. There is a lot to process when you are first diagnosed with PD," said Jane.

She Wasn't an Athlete, but She Decided Exercise Was Her Way to Tackle PD

After a few weeks of internally wrestling with demons, Jane came to a new insight. If she wanted to keep "Mr. Parkinson's" in check and not let him steamroll over her, she had better jump on the exercise band-wagon that she had read about in a pamphlet. Jane had never exercised in the "traditional" sports-enthusiast way. However, she was an equestrian. She said, "I just remembered reading that cycling was supposed to do great things for helping with PD symptoms, so I decided to try a different exercise for PD and headed straight to my first cycling class and left feeling empowered."

Seeing Courage in Others with PD Can Give You Courage

A few weeks later, Jane returned to the same class she had left feeling defeated. She had a new perspective. She explained, "When I took the class, most people were older, and I was in my 50s. And I just wasn't comfortable at first. And so, I had to step back and reboot myself. I did research about how exercise makes a major difference for PWPD. And then, when I returned to the class, I took the time to meet each person and hear all their stories. And I so admired their courage. Each of them was so brave. And it changed me. Seeing their courage in life gave me courage for my upcoming journey with PD."

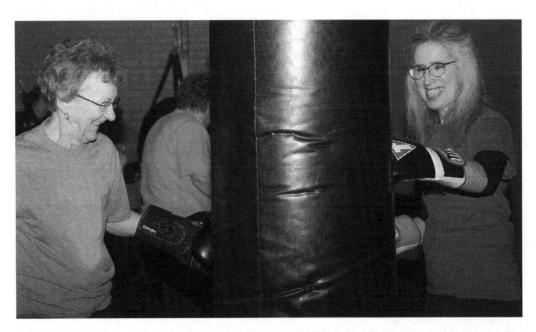

Jane Collison (right is boxing with Linda O'Hair (left) in a Rock Steady Boxing Class. Jane's PD Exercise Coctail Plan™ is called Martini —Shaken' it UP!" and includes Neuro Cycle, Rock Steady Boxing (RSB), Total Healthworks' (THW) Total Parkinson's, and strenght training.

Photo by Laraine Davis

Exercise Has Made a Huge Difference in Her Quality of Life

When Jane became my client, she was already an avid exerciser. When we sat down to map out her PD Exercise Cocktail Plan™, I first asked, "What's your favorite cocktail?" Jane answered, "A martini, shaken of course." Her PD Exercise Cocktail Plan™ is called "PD Martini—Shaken' it UP!" and included neuro-cycle, Rock Steady Boxing (RSB), Total Healthworks' (THW) Total Parkinson's, and progressive strength training.

Jane comes from a family of doctors, so it isn't surprising that one of her brothers, an MD, told her to get checked for PD. Given her family background, Jane's goal during her PD journey has been to keep her medications low—she didn't want the side effects that occur with various medicines, and she has worked with her neurologist to use exercise to keep her medications as low as possible. Jane still views exercise as her job, and she knows she has slowed her disease progression through her daily PD workouts. She is happy with what the right combination of medicine and exercise has done for her over the past eight years.

"I feel like I'm bragging every time I go to my neurologist's office. I feel that I have slowed down the progression of my disease. I've kept my medication to a minimum," said Jane. "You know, I am thankful for medication and DBS, but I have not taken the steps up that I feel I would have taken if I had not been exercising. And exercise truly has made such a difference in my quality of life." Jane also talks about how she immediately feels her symptoms worsen when she doesn't exercise because of a schedule conflict. "I get stiffer, I have more tremors. I notice a big difference even when I stop for just a few days," she said.

Change Your Cocktail as Your Life or Schedule Changes

Jane works out six days a week, sometimes twice daily, depending on her schedule. She has been one of those people who thrive on exercise—for a PWPD who started as a non-athlete, it's impressive. However, she can also change her exercise schedule and adjust her PD exercise cocktail when necessary for her life's schedule. One thing that we changed about her plan was treadmill training. She didn't naturally gravitate toward it, but she does travel, and it is something that she can do when she's on the road. It's also one of the science-proven exercises and is perfect for people who can use the treadmill. Once Jane incorporated treadmill training into her program, she was surprised that she liked it and gets a great workout. Jane also likes that she can take this workout with her when she travels so that she doesn't have to miss her training.

Another fun exercise item we added to her program, for when Jane is short on time, is a workout combining the treadmill with weights—a circuit. She spends several minutes on the treadmill, switches to the weight machines, and then returns to the treadmill. You can incorporate these types of workouts into your plan when you sit down and design them with a physical therapist or a PD exercise professional.

PD Brings Out Courage in People

"Courageous" is a word that Jane used to describe the people she met early in her PD journey. Now, after eight years of fighting her disease, Jane has become one of those courageous PWPD, and she is also a huge advocate for other PWPD in her community. I asked her what she would tell a PWPD who was thinking about exercising, or what she would say to a person who had just been diagnosed with the disease. What motivates her to keep working out? Jane admitted, "Seeing the heroes. There are a lot of brave PWPD here in the gym every day. And the encouragement you get from them—knowing firsthand how hard it is to move your body when you have PD. And seeing PWPD keep at it every day. It's something to celebrate! Everyone keeps a sense of humor, and they bring enthusiasm with them to share even when they know it's damn hard. I've met so many heroes."

SPARX Trials Have Fueled a Revolution in PD Research and Treatment

In the early 2000's, treadmill researchers were primarily interested in looking at the gait movement in PWPD. It was still very early in the exploration decade of PD exercise. The breakthrough in treadmill aerobic endurance training was SPARX2, which we discussed in Chapter 2. In an article by Maria Cohut of *Medical News Today*, the then study author Professor Corcos, PhD, (now SPARX3 lead investigator) said, "The earlier in the disease that you intervene, the more likely it is you can prevent the progression of the disease." He added, "We've delayed worsening of symptoms for six months. [In SPARX2 trial] whether we can prevent progression [of the disease] any longer than six months will require further study" (Cohut "High-Intensity"). That further study is the *Study in Parkinson's Disease of Exercise Phase 3 Clinical Trial* (Patterson et al. 2022), a $20-million-dollar clinical trial led by Professor Corcos and funded by the National Institute of Health (NIH).

Chapter 8

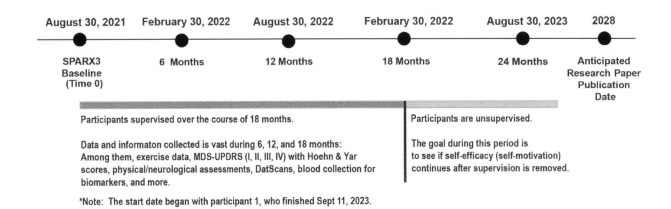

SPARX3 is a seven-year multiple site, multi-million-dollar PD treadmill exercise trial that has many phases to its endeavor. The vast amount of data and research will provide groundbreaking evidence for PD exercise.

SPARX3 Is Under Way at 24 Sites in the US and One Site in Canada

SPARX3 is being held at 24 sites in the US and one site in Canada, with 370 PWPD participating in the clinical trial. SPARX3 has opened the door to a broad population of PWPD to see whether exercise in different regions has the same results. Like SPARX2, the study has participants randomly assigned to treadmill endurance training for high intensity (80%–85% MHR) and moderate intensity (60%–65% MHR). The groups work out for thirty minutes, four times a week for eighteen months.

According to the SPARX3 Study Protocol, "The primary efficacy outcome is the MDS-UPDRS motor examination score (Part III) at twelve months. The MDS-UPDRS (Parts I–IV) is used to evaluate various aspects of PD including non-motor and motor experiences of daily living and motor complications. The MDS-UPDRS Part III is a 33-item rater-assessed evaluation of motor signs with each item rated zero to four. The motor examination score is created by summing the ratings with higher scores indicating worse motor signs. Twelve months was selected as the primary time end point as a longer-term outcome, compared to the Phase 2 trial with hypothesized trajectories of the two intervention groups based on the Phase 2 six-month changes and a sample of people with PD" (Patterson et al. 5).

SPARX3 to Test for Slowing PD Disease Progression

Dr. Jeanne Feuerstein is a neurologist and movement disorders specialist who practices at the UC Health Neurosciences Center, Anschutz Medical Campus, in Aurora, Colorado. She is a study neurologist and co-investigator for the SPARX3 trial. In an interview with *Parkinson's News Today*, she explained, "What I always say to my patients is I can give you medications that will make you function as well as you can, but the reason I'm doing it is so you can exercise. That's the key for you to actually modify the progression of the disease" (Smith "Can Exercise"). That is the focus of this study—to determine the effect of high-intensity treadmill endurance exercise in slowing the progression of PD.

SPARX3 Looks at Dopamine Uptake, Walking Speed, Blood-Derived Biomarkers, and More

SPARX 3 began on August 30, 2021, and the exercise portion of the study will conclude on July 31, 2027, while the estimated study conclusion date is July 31, 2028. Study teams closely supervise the exercise groups. For example, investigators evaluate participants' heart rates as they work out to ensure they remain in the appropriate exercise intensity range (Patterson et al. 5).

> *What I always say to my patients is I can give you medications that will make you function as well as you can, but the reason I'm doing it is so you can exercise . . . That's the key for you to actually modify the progression of the disease.*
>
> **- Dr. Jeanne Feuerstein**

The study is assessing much more than whether high-intensity exercise is superior to a moderate workout at delaying the progression of the of the disease. The study is also evaluating: "(1) whether there is a reduction in the percent decline of the striatal dopamine transporter binding at 12 months; (2) whether the progression of motor symptoms is attenuated when they continue to perform endurance treadmill exercise training at 18 months; and (3) the effects of endurance exercise training on ambulatory mobility, daily walking activity, cardiorespiratory fitness, quality of life, cognition, time to initiate dopaminergic therapy and dose of dopaminergic medication, blood-derived biomarkers of inflammation, and neurotrophic factors at 12 and 18 months" (Patterson et al. 3). In other aspects of the research, the study is collecting participants' genetic data and assessing whether genetics might play a role in each patient's response to exercise.

PD Can Descend Upon You Like a Dark Cloud, and It's Tough to Get Out from Underneath It

Getting diagnosed with PD during the midst of COVID-19 was genuinely tragic for Joe Mende. A double-decker depression sandwich is how Joe felt about the two events. The fact that he was only forty made the pill much harder to swallow. A big, dark cloud descended upon Joe, and it was not easy to get out from underneath it.

Chapter 8

SPARX3 would ultimately help him get back on track. Joe explained, "I wasn't working out much to begin with and, in general, my overall mood was not the best." But Joe, a former personal trainer and physical education teacher who lives in Chicago, felt the program would be right up his alley when he initially heard about it from his neurologist.

The SPARX3 Trial Helped Him Break Free of PD's Dark Grasp

The SPARX3 trial was a turning point for Joe. Being a part of SPARX3 brought accountability back into his life, and he thrived on being accountable to someone. Joe said, "The routine of exercising on the treadmill four times a week gave me confidence. And working out helped me shed thirty pounds of COVID-19 weight. So, it's been good. I haven't had any injuries, which is important. And, while I need and enjoy routine in my life, what is most crucial to me is to see progress. And I've had that on so many levels with SPARX3."

Exercise Has Improved Joe's Symptoms so He Can Perform on Stage with Ease Again

Joe has been a musician since the age of fourteen, and being diagnosed with PD made playing the trombone more challenging because of his tremor. In addition, being a performer on stage with PD symptoms made Joe incredibly self-conscious while playing. "Every time I took the stage, I found it difficult to focus on the music because I was also focusing on how to hide my tremors," shared Joe. "Exercising not only instilled confidence back in me to continue doing the things I love but also helped manage some of my symptoms. With my symptoms more under control, I can now enjoy what I love to do with the people I care about the most."

He Wishes There Was Another Trial to Join Because It's Been the Best Thing He Has Ever Done for His PD

Now that Joe is approaching the end of the trial, he wishes there was another one to join. But he sees his participation as a way to give back to the PD community—something he feels strongly about now.

I asked him if he was glad that he participated in SPARX3. He answered, "Yeah, for sure—100%. I'm glad I did it because, looking back, I was more depressed than I realized. If I hadn't done this, I don't know what it would have taken to get me out of that rut. I'm not much of a cardio guy, but this has taught me a lot about consistency with exercising. It's been good, and I love the way I feel. I'm probably in the best shape I've been in my entire life. It feels good to be healthy."

If You Are Undecided About Doing a Clinical Trial, Make the Decision and Get Into One. You'll be glad You Did

Joe has always believed in the power of exercise. It's why he chose his career path in exercise science and health. He explained, "I've always believed exercise can create change in so many things, and that has been my guiding principle throughout my life. So, the fact that exercise can help manage Parkinson's symptoms is not hard for me to understand at all. I believe it. And I also hope if anyone is sitting on the fence about doing a clinical trial, you jump off and get into one. Participating in this study has been the best decision I've ever made. And from what I understand, SPARX3 will help a lot of PWPD in the future. So, I'm so glad I was a part of it."

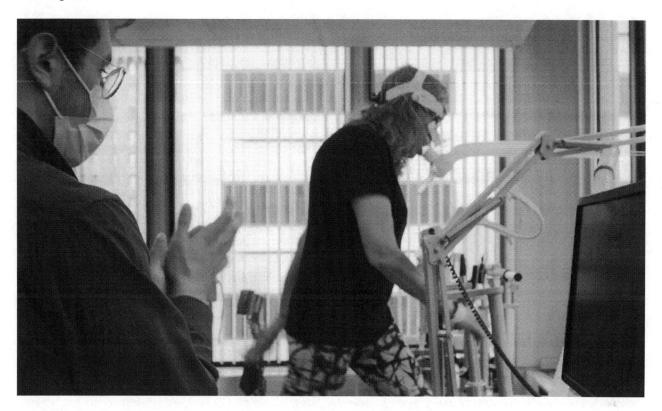

A researcher encourages a participant in the SPARX3 trial, following the protocol.

Lead Investigator, Professor Daniel Corcos Talks about SPARX3

I interviewed Professor Daniel Corcos, who explained that SPARX3 would be a significant study on PD exercise with an in-depth analysis of what occurs in the brain during high-intensity exercise. A significant number of the world's leading posture, gait, and balance experts make up the SPARX3 team. Professor Corcos shared what they will be looking for in the research. "We are looking at scans of the dopamine transporter that people get with a DaTscan (dopamine transporter scan). And if it's positive, you will likely have the disease. So, it's still not definitive, but it does provide one more confirmatory piece of information. At the end of the first twelve months, we have another DaTscan. The DaTscan looks at how dopamine is binding in the striatum. It is possible that the baseline will be one value, and at twelve months, it will be different between the two intensity groups [the high-intensity and moderate-intensity exercise groups]. And if we find that, our paper will be submitted to a prestigious journal since there would be clear biological evidence that the intensity of endurance exercise is a key variable in whether exercise is neuroprotective and affects how dopamine binds in the striatum. And this would be very exciting news."

Chapter 8

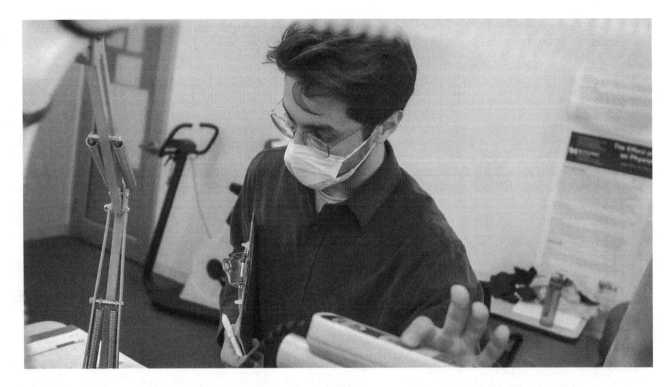

The research results from the SPARX3 study will produce key information for the future of PD exercise.

SPARX3 Will Produce an Enormous Amount of Data about PD Exercise

SPARX3 postulates a difference of 3.5 points between the high-intensity and the moderate-intensity groups (MDS-UPDRS Part III motor signs). If the study results in this number and it is statistically significant, then the SPARX3 team will have achieved the study's goal. But Professor Corcos says that regardless of the points difference, the amount of data SPARX3 will produce is enormous. "We will have over 740 DaTscans to analyze. And so that's one area that I'll be looking for financial support in. And we're going to write lots of papers—about how exercise improves speed, stride length, and gait symmetry. The team will use what is called an 'opal tracking system' with participants. Five markers go on the arms, legs, and back so they will be monitored. The participants will do the six-minute walk, and the markers will pick up sensitive gait measures. For example, PWPD have asymmetry between the arms, and exercise helps improve turning velocity [PWPD require time to slow down before turning along with more steps to complete a turn while turning more slowly than those without the disease]. And so, we're also going to have a set of papers on how all these aspects of gait improve or stay constant. Remember, if you stay constant [the disease doesn't progress] over two years, you've come out ahead with PD."

SPARX3 Will Also Look at PWPD Activity Levels After They Exercise

That isn't all the study is going to investigate. The burning questions are, "Does PD exercise increase activity, keep activity the same in PWPD, or decrease activity? How many people want to go home and nap after that high-intensity workout versus feeling ready to go out and conquer the world?" As Professor Corcos explained to me, "To do this, participants wear activity monitors called 'ActivPal' for one week every month. These activity monitors allow the investigators of SPARX3 to continuously track activity of participants and determine if the treadmill exercise leads to altered patterns of physical activity during the day and sleep patterns at night. I will need to raise funds for several post-doctoral positions to analyze this extensive data set in a timely fashion. In addition, other teams will be looking into hormones, neurotrophic factors, blood biochemistry, and cardiopulmonary assessments. Does the 80-to 85-MHR group increase peak oxygen consumption (VO2 peak), while the other group doesn't? So now we can ask, what is driving this increase in VO2 peak? If you can take in more oxygen and transport more oxygen around the body in the bloodstream, then the oxygen gets to the brain, and this is very beneficial."

Time will tell what impact this study will have on the treatment of PD; however, it is likely to increase the data supporting intense exercise in the treatment of PD.

- Professor Daniel M. Corcos, PhD

SPARX3 Will Bring Exciting Advancement to PD Exercise

"Time will tell what impact this study will have on the treatment of PD; however, it is likely to increase the data supporting intense exercise in the treatment of PD," said Professor Corcos. He would like the clinical trial to wrap up sooner than the projected completion date of July 31, 2028. However, a great deal of data from all the different testing sites will have to be evaluated, and then, twenty or more papers will need to be written, based on the information compiled during the course of the study and post-study analysis. Nevertheless, the SPARX3 website sparx3pd.com will post key results as soon as they are announced and will explain how they contribute to the understanding of PD exercise.

Dr Alberts and Cleveland Clinic Join SPARX3 Trials

Dr. Alberts and his colleagues at the Cleveland Clinic are currently part of the SPARX3 study and one of the 25 study sites. Like the other sites, the investigators have enrolled newly diagnosed PWPD who have not yet started PD medication. Participants have been and will be randomly assigned to eighteen months of treadmill walking and/or running for thirty minutes four times a week at either high intensity (80%–85% MHR) or moderate intensity (60%–65% MHR).

Higher-Intensity Exercise Is Expected to Yield Greater Neuroprotection

In a recent *Cleveland Clinic Consult QD online* article titled *SPARX3 Intensifies Efforts Toward a Specific Exercise Prescription in Parkinson's Disease* (SPARX3 Intensifies), Dr. Alberts said, "Both studies [CYCLE-II and SPARX3] work from the hypothesis that neuroprotection is likely to be triggered by high-intensity exercise involving a relatively high heart rate" (SPARX3 Intensifies).

As with the cycle studies, the primary goal of the treadmill study is to measure the change in PD motor symptoms in participants at the twelve-month marker, as measured by the Movement Disorders Society–modified Unified Parkinson Disease Rating Scale (MDS–UPDRDS). The 1980s-developed UPDRS and MDS-UPDRS (early 2000s) are tools to measure the severity and progression of Parkinson disease (Unified Parkinson's). There will also be secondary measures of motor symptoms at eighteen months as well as a measure of changes in dopaminergic activity, walking capacity, cognitive function, fitness, activity, and quality of life at both twelve and eighteen months.

Both CYCLE-II and SPARX3 Will Help Refine Exercise Prescriptions

Dr. Alberts says the studies' results should provide much-needed guidance on what level of exercise is therapeutically beneficial in PD. He states, "These two multi-site clinical trials are expected to help identify a patient-specific exercise prescription for PD. The great thing is that PWPD tend to adhere highly to their therapies. In this case, we need to determine the effective exercise therapy they should adhere to."

SPARX3 Looks at More Diverse Representation across the Nation

Dr. Alberts adds that SPARX3 is also notable because it has a particular emphasis on outreach to communities that are traditionally underrepresented in PD clinical trials. In the *Cleveland Clinic Consult QD* online article, he noted, "We expect this study to have a patient sample that's much more diverse and representative—racially, ethnically, socioeconomically, across the board— than many clinical trials" (SPARX3 Intensifies). The SPARX3 study is expected to be completed in mid-2028. Completion of the Cleveland Clinic-led study of high-intensity cycling in PD is expected in early 2024.

Treadmill Aerobic Endurance Exercise Training for PWPD

Treadmill training is an aerobic endurance workout for PWPD who are not experiencing balance or gait issues. The definition of gait is how a person walks. As PD progresses, some individuals slowly lose their innate walking stride to the point that they shuffle in small steps.

Treadmill Training Requires Building a Cardio Base

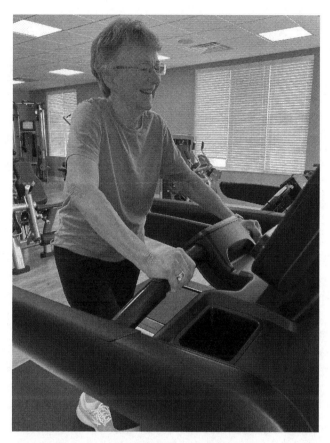

Linda O'Hair is taking time to learn the buttons on the treadmill machine before starting her workout. Each participant knows where the emergency stop button is located and can immediately stop the treadmill for any reason.

As shown with SPARX2 trial results in Chapter 2, treadmill training helps slow disease progression. Just like neuro-cycling, you need to build an aerobic base for six to eight weeks if you are starting from a sedentary activity level or getting back to exercise after taking time off. Aerobic base-building information is described in Chapter 6.

Once you have built that base, you will want to find your heart-rate zones to determine what is your 80%–85% MHR (see Chapter 6). From there, if necessary, you can work in intervals (short bursts of work followed by short segments of rest) to increase your time at that high-intensity range.

There are different ways to achieve this on the treadmill:

- Through speed
- Through adding resistance by altering treadmill incline
- Through a combination of speed and resistance

Gait training and treadmill exercise training serve two different purposes and different audiences. Gait training is for PWPD that have issues with gait who need to work with a physical therapist to improve their walking abilities through slow treadmill training. Treadmill exercise is for PWPD who have no restrictions and can walk or jog freely on the treadmill.

Learn to Use the Treadmill So You Can Safely Operate It

It is crucial to have someone show you how to use a treadmill machine and all its buttons. Learn how to use the speed buttons and how they adjust up and down until you are comfortable and can safely work the controls—especially while the treadmill is moving. Most importantly, know where the emergency stop button is located on the machine. That way, you can immediately stop the treadmill for any reason. There should always be an emergency stop cord you can pull or even hook on to you for extra safety measures. We want to prevent any falls from occurring.

Follow the SPARX3 Workout for the Treadmill

The workout used by the SPARX3 research trial is unstructured; it is up to the individual to determine how they want to reach the target of 80% MHR. You warm up for five minutes. Then, you adjust the machine's speed, resistance, or both to get to your target heart rate zone. You work out at this pace for thirty minutes (take recoveries—slow down the speed or incline on the treadmill and let your heart-rate come down) when needed and cool down for five minutes, then do muscle stretching exercises after you get off the machine.

Treadmill Classes for Those Who Can Jog or Have No Gait or Balance Issues

Currently, there are no treadmill classes specifically for PWPD. However, if you are in Stage 1 of your PD journey, there is no reason you could not attend a non-PD treadmill class. If you try one of these classes, here is what you can expect. A class would start with a warm-up, preparing the body for the workout. The remainder of the class will be divided into "blocks of work" for specified periods. Many of these classes would have a theme with an objective to meet for each day. Perhaps the theme would be "The Hills Are Alive" on the day you go, and it will be a strength and conditioning "hill climbing" workout that day. Of course, your objective will always be to try to hit 80% MHR for as much of the class as possible—regardless of the class objective for the day.

Workouts Are Divided into Blocks to Enable You to Tackle Them One at a Time—It Feels More Manageable

The instructor will explain how the class will proceed with each work block. For instance, block one may have five minutes of hill repeats. The instructor may tell you to add resistance, jog up a hill for thirty seconds, and then walk down the hill for thirty seconds, and repeat five times for that block of work. An instructor will organize the class this way, with some blocks longer and some shorter. It will be up to you to determine how much resistance to add to get your heart rate to the target max of 80%. It will take time to figure these things out, but once you start adjusting the resistance and the speed, you will quickly see where it places your heart rate (or PRE). You should go to one of these classes early and get assistance from the instructor if you have any questions that you want answered before the class begins.

Treadmill Training Case Studies
Rhonda Foulds (Justin, Texas)

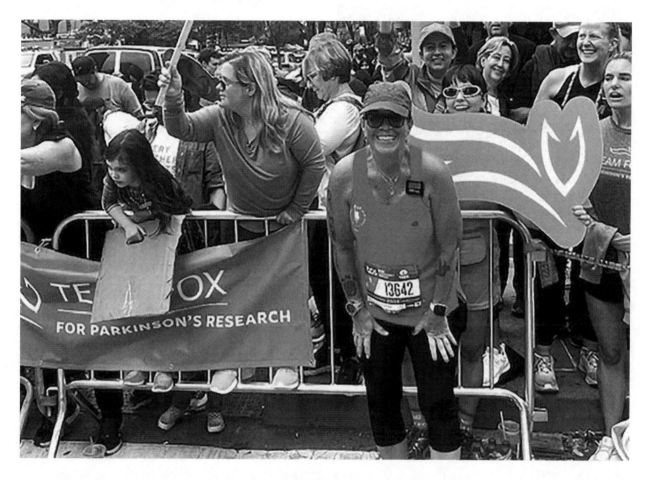

Rhonda Foulds takes a photo with the Michael J. Fox Parkinson's support team cheering on the runners at the 2022 New York City Marathon.

PD Was in Control of Her Life at Age 40

Rhonda's body had physically deteriorated to needing a wheelchair five years after she was diagnosed with PD at age 35. Rhonda was 40 when she was rolled into her neurologist's office in a wheelchair on the day she would be "turned on" after Deep Brain Stimulation Surgery (DBS). The doctor turned on a handheld controller to be used by the patient to turn the DBS system on and off. The doctor then asked Rhonda to get up and walk and perform movements. "I remember the neurologist said, 'You need to get out of the wheelchair, lose weight, and start exercising. It would be best if you did more for yourself,'" recalled Rhonda. What that doctor said greatly impacted her fight with PD. He kicked her butt right out of that wheelchair, and she never returned to it.

Chapter 8

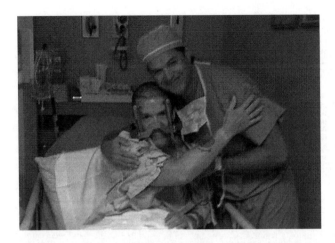

Rhonda Foulds, left, with Dr. J. Michael Desaloms, Neurosurgeon, MD, after her Deep Brain Stimulation Surgery in Dallas, Texas, in 2004. She was 40 years old and one of the youngest people at the time to have DBS.

Looking Back, She Couldn't Believe She Had Let PD Drag Her So Far Down

Rhonda continued, "I had gained a lot of weight in five years because I had stopped exercising and sat in a wheelchair, but I couldn't believe he said that to my face. He pissed me off." Angry, she turned to him and said, "How can you know what I'm going through? I'm sick! How can you be mean to me? How can you say those things?" But he just repeated what he had said and reemphasized that if Rhonda wanted to manage her PD, this was what she needed to do. Rhonda thought hard for a moment, "I was a quasi-athlete before this. Not a great one, but I don't want to live my life in a wheelchair.

Having the Courage to Take Control of Her Life through Exercise

When Rhonda got home, she started walking. Her son was in the U.S. Marine Corps. He came home on leave one day and saw her walking. And he asked, "Mom, when was the last time you ran?" She answered, "It's been ten years."

He said, "Well, let's try to run from this pole to the next pole." And that's how she got started. Just that little bit of running felt so good to her because she was claiming back her life from PD. And on the way home that day, there was a billboard that said, "Join us for a 5K run." She saw that she had three months to prepare for the race. And she thought, "I'm going to run that 5K." And she did. It was the first timed race she had ever run in her life—and she had PD. And everything just picked up from there.

Having Early-Onset PD Was Not Something Believable

Let's back up to see how Rhonda ended up here. Before PD, she was a welder for an aerospace company in upstate New York. Her husband still works for that company, and she has since retired. In 1996, they transferred to a branch in Justin, Texas, close to the Oklahoma border. Now, Rhonda was just a casual runner in her youth. She never even timed or tracked her distances. Rhonda just liked to run to keep in shape, and running made her feel good. After they moved to Texas, she got "a wild hair" and decided to train for the White Rock Marathon in Dallas. She started a training program. Sometimes her husband would follow her in the car as she trained. One day he noticed Rhonda was dragging her right foot. Rhonda also noticed that she started to trip more often and fall because of that foot. But she didn't think anything of it. But when she got a tremor in her pinkie finger and jaw, she decided to go to the neurologist.

She Thought It Was Just Overtraining—It Wasn't

"I thought they were going to tell me I was overtraining, but it was the first time I ever heard the word 'Parkinson's' regarding me," said Rhonda. "I mean, I knew about it. My grandfather had it, and my father had it. But I did not believe the neurologist when he told me I had it."

A Diagnosis of PD Sent Rhonda Spiraling

Rhonda went to see several specialists to confirm her diagnosis. She didn't believe them when they said PD. However, all of them agreed that Rhonda did have PD. And upon diagnosis, Rhonda says, she made the biggest mistake of her life. She stopped exercising altogether. She became depressed and went physically and mentally downhill at a rapid pace. The situation spiraled out of control until finally she was in a wheelchair and needed DBS surgery. She thanks her neurologist, who set her straight and woke her up from a life-threatening situation. Rhonda said, "I was wallowing in my pity party and can only thank my doctor for waking me up. PD was killing me at the age of 40."

After Rhonda victoriously completed her first "billboard sign" 5K run, as a woman with PD, she kept running 5K and 10K races. She then decided to train for the original marathon that she never got to run because she was diagnosed with PD—the White Rock Marathon in Dallas, Texas.

How Rhonda Found Information on Marathon Running for PWPD

You may wonder how Rhonda figured out how to be a marathon runner as a PWPD. She searched the internet for anything she could find on Parkinson's and running. She found an author named John Ball, another PWPD (the next story in this book), who had written a book titled *Living Well, Running Hard: Lessons Learned from Living with Parkinson's Disease*. Rhonda bought his book and read it. When she finished the book, she thought, "If this guy can do it, I can do it." Then she called him, and he personally advised her on how to train. A friendship was born. She has stayed in contact with John throughout the years.

Rhonda prepared an eighteen-week training plan for her first marathon. She started in December and built up to twenty-mile runs on the weekends. Rhonda explained, "That's how I trained. Smaller runs during the week with a long twenty-mile run on the weekend. But I did the majority of my running on the treadmill." Rhonda did most of her training on the treadmill because the temperature outside in Texas in the summer is so hot.

Chapter 8

One Marathon Was Enough—Or So She Thought

Rhonda completed her first marathon with fierce determination and intense joy. Afterward, Rhonda felt she never wanted to run another twenty-six miles again. However, Medtronic Medical Device Company contacted Rhonda to run in their *Be a Global Hero Event*—at a Twin Cities Marathon in Minnesota. Rhonda had ten months to prepare for her second marathon. While in Minnesota, she caught the marathon bug and decided this was something she wanted to keep doing in her life. She started running three to four marathons a year.

Never Count Yourself Out—Find a Reason to Keep Getting Up and Fight PD Everyday

Rhonda, who was in a wheelchair at the beginning of her battle with PD, has run 110 marathons—and this doesn't count her 5Ks, 10Ks, and half-marathons. And this is what she will tell you about her experience with PD: "Never count yourself out. I've run 110 marathons with PD—because I never ran a race until after I got PD. And that's not a bragging thing. I'm just a middle-aged, old lady. I'm 60 years old with three grown boys and grandchildren. Who would have thought that I would be able to run the Boston Marathon ten times? So, you never know what you're capable of until you try to push the envelope. And when it comes to PD, it's imperative to find out what you can accomplish daily. I feel that's the one thing that makes me excited to get out of bed every day, even with PD, to see what I can do. So that's what I encourage everyone to do. Find something that excites you and gets you out of bed, and do it."

Exercise Has Kept Her in a High-Functioning State for Twenty-Five Years

Rhonda credits exercise with her ability to function for so long and so well while having PD. She says, "After twenty-five years with Parkinson's, people still don't realize when they meet me that I have PD. So that's crazy. I was one of the youngest people in Dallas to have DBS, and they knew I had to continue to exercise and push myself. And I'm lucky that I had my surgeon who wanted to do my surgery while I was young. Back then they didn't like to do DBS until much older ages—over 60. And I think that is why my surgeon was so tough on me. It would have been a waste in so many ways if I hadn't made the most of that surgery. My quality of life has been and is fantastic. And I can thank my surgeon, myself, my husband, and my kids for making that happen."

Exercise Needs to Become as Much a Part of Your Daily Routine as Brushing Your Teeth

"I just look at exercise as part of my daily routine," said Rhonda. "It's no different than brushing my teeth or anything else. I must do it every single day." Rhonda says that she has people calling her all the time. Unfortunately, it's usually the spouse of somebody with PD, and the person on the other end of the line

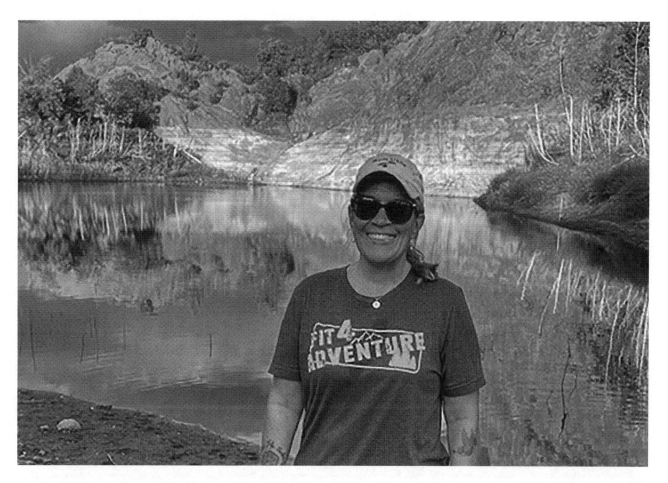

Rhonda looks at exercise as part of her daily routine. She says, " It's no different than brushing my teeth or anything else. I must do it every single day."

will say, "Will you talk to my husband? He won't exercise, and I'm worried about his health and condition because I know he is getting worse." And Rhonda will tell the person on the phone that unless the PWPD calls himself and talks to her, nothing is going to change. But, if the person on the other end can get the spouse to call, she will be happy to speak to him. Sadly, the spouse with PD never calls Rhonda back.

People Are Around Us Everywhere—You Just Have to Open Your Eyes and Look

Rhonda also has people routinely ask her, "How do you continue to run like this?" And she responds, "Well, I've had such incredible benefits from exercise. Why would I not do it? Exactly why would I stop? If I stopped, I would regress to where I started: in a wheelchair. No thanks." Rhonda has a female friend who is 79 years old and inspires Rhonda. They run together twice a week. Her friend doesn't have PD, but ran the 2022 Athens Classic Greek Marathon in Greece. "There are inspiring people all around us, every day," said Rhonda. "All you have to do is open your eyes and look. You will see them right in front of you."

Chapter 8

Treadmill Training Case Studies
John Ball (Los Angeles, California)

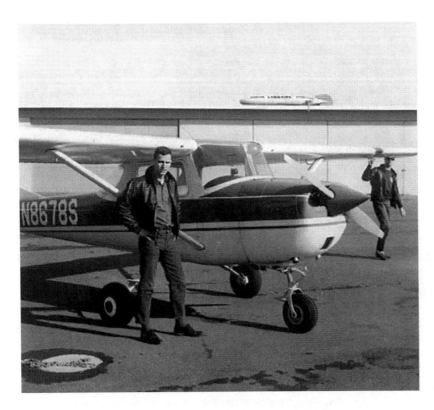

John Ball was a U.S. Navy pilot who thought he had the world on a string. He didn't think anything could stop him. This photo of John (left) was taken at Paine Field in Everett, Washington, in 1966.

One Misdiagnosis After the Other Caused Quite a Few Scares

Imagine being misdiagnosed with myasthenia gravis (a chronic, autoimmune, neuromuscular disease that causes weakness in the skeletal muscles), blood circulation problems, a brain tumor, and even having surgery on your piriformis muscle when, in fact, you had PD all along. But in 1983, it was difficult to diagnose someone who was only 38 years old as having PD, and John Ball just happened to be the lucky guy doctors kept misdiagnosing.

Prior to his diagnosis, the former U.S. Navy pilot felt he had the world on a string. "Yeah, nothing could stop me," John thought, until PD brought his life to a screeching halt. John was 27 when he first started having strange symptoms, and he said, "It brought me down a few notches, let's face it. I had to take myself a little less seriously."

Crippling Symptoms Made It Impossible to Do His Normal Activities

John got up for his morning run and noticed that his foot turned under, making it difficult to walk and too painful to run. John explained, "When I tried to run, my toes on my left foot would turn under, making it impossible to run." He didn't know it then, but he had dystonia (contractions resulting in twisting parts of the body). He couldn't run for the next eleven years. He said, "I was suffering from a distorting foot but had no tremors. And so, there were no cardinal signs of PD. I still have no tremors fifty years later. I still have dystonia, though."

PD Was Taking Away His Abilities, One Thing at a Time

John was diagnosed with PD in 1983. He explained how miraculous it was once he started taking PD medication. As his symptoms progressed, he had gone from playing softball in the outfield to second base to pitcher. And finally, he was reduced to catching the ball behind the plate, and he couldn't throw it back to the pitcher's mound without bouncing it. However, after he took his first tablet of Sinemet (a PD medicine approved by the FDA in 1975), by the second inning he could throw the ball back to the pitcher without bouncing.

Little Yellow Magic Beans Take Away Symptoms so He Can Run again After Eleven Years

John called the little yellow pills his "magic beans," because he suddenly felt normal again after eleven years. Being able to throw a ball again wasn't the only thing that changed. The medicine enabled John to run again. It had been more than a decade since he was able to run. Now he knew he had PD, but he wasn't going to let that diagnosis stop him from running. He was going to make up for lost time.

John's first goal in 1983 was to get through a 5K. Once he accomplished this goal, he set his sights on a half-marathon. His goal after that was to run the 1996 Los Angeles Marathon. And he did. Eventually—get ready for this—John ran the Los Angeles Marathon sixteen times in a row.

Team Parkinson Is Born and Helps Many Achieve Their Dreams

A friend of John's, Mary Yost (who also has PD), saw him run in the 1999 Los Angeles Marathon and decided she wanted to run it too. In 2000 Mary started Team Parkinson, an official non-profit PD charity organization for the Los Angeles Marathon, after she ran her first marathon. John and his wife, Edna, joined Team Parkinson and have helped countless PWPD run or walk marathons over the past twenty-two years.

Over the years, Team Parkinson has raised over $3 million dollars to support the PD community in Los Angeles. John decided to help others with PD learn to run and wrote a book called *Living Well, Running Hard: Lessons Learned from Living with Parkinson's Disease*. John said, "I think the problem is that most people stop thinking of themselves as athletes once they are adults. If you're in your 30s or 40s and don't get diagnosed until you're 50 or later, taking up sports again is tough, so you've already started at a deficit. Beginning to exercise again seems challenging to PWPD. However, I think exercise is essential for treating PD—absolutely. You've got to find what you like so that you'll continue to do it. If you don't like it, you won't do it and you will be fighting with yourself."

John Has Had PD for Fifty Years and Is Still Running Half-Marathons at Age 78

John has had PD for fifty years. He is living proof of what high-intensity exercise can do for a person with PD. He said, "How many people do you see walking around like me after fifty years with PD? It's a very rare sight, right? PD is a degenerative disease, yet here I am." He ran his first marathon at age 51 in 1996 and his last half-marathon at age 78 in 2022. And he doesn't seem to be slowing down any time soon.

The Truth, the Whole Truth, and Nothing but the Truth

I asked John what he would tell someone recently diagnosed with PD. He answered, "Well, here is the truth of the matter. Everyone with PD will have to face the reality that the less they do, the less they can do. On the flip side, the more you do, the more you'll be able to do. So again, find something you love, do it frequently, and as hard as possible. That's my basic, core philosophy. I will go as long as possible and as hard as possible. And then I'm going to do more."

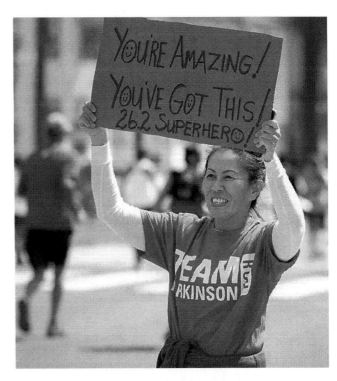

Tracy Mei Wong of Team Parkinson cheers on her team at the 2019 Los Angeles Marathon.

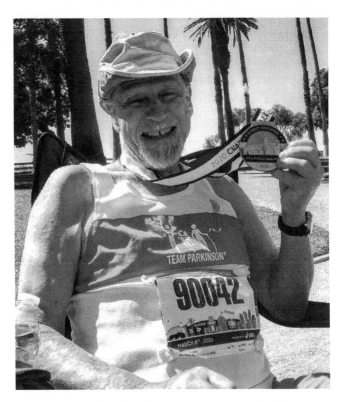

John Ball is an inspiration. He has had PD for fifty years and yet in 2022, he ran the LA half-marathon in Los Angeles, California, at 78 years old.

PD Teaches Lessons We Didn't Know We Needed to Learn

John is motivated by a group of friends that he has acquired through PD. If John's group gets together to walk five miles on a Sunday morning, he joins them; he never wants to disappoint them. He explained, "I will be there regardless of how I feel because they get something from it. And PD has taught me how to be a good friend to people. I wasn't particularly good at being friends as a kid. So, I appreciate now being able to energize other people."

You Have to Push Yourself Beyond What You Think You Can Do

Many people I have interviewed have shared how PD has made them better people than they were previously. John shared that this was also true in his case. "I was an arrogant asshole most of my youth because things came too easy to me. And then, with PD, everything stopped coming easy. PD is mean. It is the great teacher of humility that helped me enormously. Without it, I never would have created an organization to help others." John believes he is a better man today than he would have been without PD.

Everyone Should Work Out, With or Without a Disease

John and his wife, Edna, work out together performing progressive strength training. John believes exercise benefits everyone, not just those with neurodegenerative diseases. He also believes it's not enough just to know you need to exercise. One must be diligent about it. John said, "Exercise needs to be taxing, and you've got to push yourself beyond what you think you can do. So many people set limitations on their performance irrespective of what they can achieve. We can all work beyond what we think we can, and that is when a coach can help us find what we're truly made of."

Find Your Hero and Let Them Inspire and Guide You

John's mother-in-law passed away from PD. She was a Holocaust survivor and first got PD symptoms in her 40s. She was diagnosed at age 48. She was John's hero because she lived with PD and survived for forty years in the most challenging times. He mentioned how important it is to have a hero to look up to, and to gain strength from their shared experiences when you struggle through difficult times with PD. He explained, "I've been so fortunate to continue to build a community of people around me that supports me. And in numerous ways, not just with physical support, but with their friendship and desire to see me succeed. It's been a real blessing in my life."

Nothing Is More Important Than Your Family Standing with You on Your Journey

We talk about the PD care team a great deal. The core of that team is, of course, the family unit. John's family has played an essential role in his journey with PD. His daughter has run several marathons. His son, Dave, ran one marathon with Team Parkinson to show his support. And last year, when John ran his half-marathon at the age of 78, his daughter, Sarah, his son, Dave, and Dave's wife, Shaili ran the race with him.

The Care Partner Is the Glue That Holds It All Together

The family's glue is Edna, John's wife. John becomes very emotional when he talks about Edna—tears well up in his eyes as he speaks with love and gratitude. December of 2023 will mark the 50th wedding anniversary of this remarkable couple, who have shared a journey they could not have foreseen the day they got married.

Edna grew up in a family with PD, although she does not have PD herself. Edna was eleven years old when her mother was diagnosed with PD at the age of 48. Edna has spent her entire life caring for loved ones with PD. John said, "She's probably the world's most knowledgeable care partner. She stuck through it all and I couldn't have done it without her. Without her, we wouldn't have built this community."

You've Got to Show Up First Before You Can Help Others

John Ball has spent most of his life helping PWPD find the fire within to take charge of their own lives. You have read Rhonda Foulds' story in this book. Like countless others, she searched the internet, found John Ball, and contacted him directly for help when her life was in crisis—PD was crushing her. And John helped her flip her world around to smash PD through exercise. I asked John how many people he thought he had helped. He said, "I've helped many people by helping myself. But you must help yourself first so that you can help others. If you're not there, you can't make a difference. So, you've got to show up and take care of yourself first, and then you can help others."

CHAPTER 9

Parkinson's Science-Proven Exercise: Progressive Strength Training

"Resilience is the ability to transform yourself as you move through adversity or painful experiences, to grow stronger, more flourishing, and more mentally free."

- NFL Veteran Steve Gleason, ALS Team Gleason Non-Profit

He Was Just Diagnosed With PD and Kept Falling All the Time

Kim Beisser (age 72), CEO of Beisser Lumber Company, Grimes, Iowa, fell fifty-three times between December 20, 2021, and September 2022. Kim has what's called "freezing of gait."

When PWPD freeze, they are stuck to the floor and unable to produce steps to start walking forward, or they stop entirely in the middle of walking and can't move in any direction. When this happens, it's natural to panic because no matter what they do, they can't move, and a fall usually occurs. Kim came to his first personal treadmill and cycle training session using a cane and wearing a protective headband. After hearing his story and looking at the photos of his head with gashes and bumps, I didn't blame him. He had experienced a crash course in extreme PD.

88% of Adults 55+ Are at Risk for Sarcopenia (Muscle Mass Loss)—One in Five PWPD Have a Severe Case

Nothing on the CT scans the neurologist had ordered showed anything to explain Kim's excessive falling. My suspicion was sarcopenia (severe loss of muscle mass that can lead to falling in PWPD). "Sarcopenia is a prevalent condition among older adults with PD, with severe sarcopenia being diagnosed in up to one in every five men and women . . . the role of prevention and intervention for sarcopenia in PD should be discussed. In PD, sarcopenia may represent the common downstream pathway that leads from motor and non-motor symptoms to the progressive loss of resilience, frailty, and disability" (Vetrano et al. 526). Here is the good news about sarcopenia: it's treatable, preventable, and reversible through progressive strength training.

After Training for Two Months, Kim Stopped Falling

Kim had been trying to work with me since he attended my March 2022 Parkinson's Awareness Month Event where I gave my *How to Exercise to Reduce PD Symptoms* presentation. However, he had had the Watchman procedure done (a treatment for atrial fibrillation) and needed to recover for several months before starting his PD program. Life was giving him overwhelming challenges. Since his surgery, he had been working with a physical therapist (doing the LSVT® Big program—see Chapter 5), and a personal trainer was helping him work on the movements that he was learning in the LSVT ®Big program. The continuous falling was creating fear, anxiety, and taking away his hope.

Exercise Can Give You Hope When You Understand What Is Possible

My goal was to help improve Kim's PD symptoms, lift his spirits, and give him back hope. We finally started in October 2022, with a ten-minute treadmill training session followed by ten minutes on the indoor bike. He could easily hit the target of 80 RPM from the start, which was a good sign of his ability to get results quickly. After we finished, Kim said, "This is harder than I have been doing, but I feel better just with that short amount. Thank you." Right then, we made a pact to start working his aerobic endurance sessions two times a week.

You Never Know What Little Trick Will Work to Unfreeze Someone

Over the next month, Kim continued to work diligently. Whenever he would freeze in the workout room, I would ask, "Shall we dance?" and hold my hands out like we were going to waltz. He would take them, and off we'd go. He could walk as if he'd never been frozen. The verbal interchange would get his brain thinking of something else. He would relax and laugh, which helped the freezing release. And moving forward to dance reengaged his body without him thinking about it. Kim would laugh and say, "I'm going to have to take you everywhere, so I don't have to worry about freezing anymore."

After Making Consistent Progress in Training, Kim Stopped Falling

Kim continued to make progress with the treadmill and biking, and we added thirty minutes of progressive strength training after his aerobics. As the weeks passed, we slowly added a minute or two to the cardio sessions. His stamina, movement, and stride improved. His speed on the treadmill increased. And, as happens when you exercise with the correct PD methodology, Kim stopped falling.

The month of October went by, and no falls. He didn't fall in November and was doing great. Kim was ecstatic. We added THW's Total Parkinson's class to his PD plan for additional brain work. During the cardio segment, he worked in the chair to ensure his safety and did exceptionally well with the PD-specific portion of the class. In December, he had one fall. He missed a step going down the stairs in his home. However, considering where we started, he was doing remarkably better—one fall in three months versus 53 falls in the previous ten months.

Exercise Training Kept Kim from Being in a Wheelchair

Kim had made an appointment with his neurologist, who didn't know he had been falling before starting our training. Kim hadn't seen her since his regular six-month visit. After reviewing what had happened, she sent him to a movement specialist at the University of Iowa Hospitals & Clinics for a separate consultation. Kim told the specialist everything that had happened and what steps he had taken with exercise to gain back control of his spiraling symptom. The movement specialist told Kim, "You are fortunate to have started the treadmill, bike, and strength training with your exercise coach. Because if you hadn't done that, you would be in a wheelchair by now."

He Told Him to Keep It Up in Order to Stay Out of the Wheelchair

Kim was incredibly relieved and grateful for all the work we had done. Particularly after hearing those words. The specialist also told him, "You must keep doing your exercise training because that is the only thing that will keep you from going into a wheelchair." Kim is highly motivated to work out. He always feels so much better after we've finished a session, and the stress of falling isn't at the forefront of his mind anymore.

In the classes he takes, there is music and laughter, and he enjoys seeing other PWPD. When I asked him about falling, he said, "I feel so good when I'm not falling, and I felt stronger exercising than I had before. I would share with others to exercise no matter what. And when you're walking, even though it's hard, try not to stop and think about falling or freezing."

It Is Crucial for Everyone to Maintain Muscle Mass and Strength as We Age

We have all heard the phrase "use it or lose it." Well, when it comes to muscle mass, this mantra is true. Working the muscles as we age helps maintain muscle mass and strength. When muscles are not used, they shrink. It's as simple as that. Unfortunately, muscle power (force production over time) ebbs at an even faster rate than strength. And the ability to generate power dramatically impacts a person's ability to perform activities of daily life—going up the stairs, grabbing something quickly, or moving faster through the crosswalk because the light suddenly turned yellow.

Sarcopenia Is Age-Related Loss of Muscle Mass That Effects Everyone Starting about the Age of 40

What isn't stressed enough in our culture is that from age 40, we start to lose muscle mass, function, and strength. Why is this important? This change can affect balance, gait, and a person's overall ability to perform the simple tasks of daily living. Why is this phenomenon even more critical for people with neurological diseases? Because it's a double whammy for them. One, they must fight the effects of sarcopenia, which brings on falls, fractures, and frailty. "Sarcopenia, age-associated loss of muscle mass and strength, is associated with increased risk for functional limitation, mobility decline, and mortality" (Hicks et al. 66). And two, they must fight the myriad of symptoms associated with their disease.

Chapter 9

One in Five People With PD Have Severe Sarcopenia

A 2018 observational study titled *Sarcopenia in Parkinson Disease: Comparison of Different Criteria and Association with Disease Severity* (Vetrano et al. 523-527) found that, "Sarcopenia is common in PD, with severe sarcopenia being diagnosed in one in every five patients with PD." The study stated, "Among the 210 participants (mean age 73 years; 38% women), the prevalence of sarcopenia was 28.5%—40.7% in men and 17.5%—32.5% in women. The prevalence of severe sarcopenia was 16.8%—20.0% in men and 11.3%—18.8% in women" (Vetrano et al. 523).

* * *

What isn't stressed enough in our culture is that from age 40, we start to lose muscle mass, function, and strength. Why is this important? This change can affect balance, gait, and a person's overall ability to perform the simple tasks of daily living. Why is this phenomenon even more critical for people with neurological diseases? Because it's a double whammy for them. One, they must fight the effects of sarcopenia, which brings on falls, fractures, and frailty . . . And two, they must fight the myriad of symptoms associated with their disease.

* * *

Dynapenia (Loss of Muscle Strength) Is Now on the Horizon as an Even Greater Concern for PWPD

Dynapenia is the loss of muscle strength. However, it is not caused by neurologic or muscular diseases. Dynapenia, like sarcopenia, is related to aging, and is more prevalent in females. Dynapenia reflects the overall muscle weakness of the body and indicates other health issues that could be coming down the road if left unchecked. Working to keep your muscle strength as you age will translate into good muscle quality and body functionality. It is essential to prevent yourself from getting either of these conditions, and let's talk about why.

Low Muscle Strength Affects Gait and Contributes to Falls

Several studies (Yazar et al. 1415-1421, Ozer et al. 313-320) have shown that low muscle strength goes hand in hand with poor physical performance and disability—the dreaded gait issues. We talked earlier about gait being how a person walks. Now, you may say to yourself, "Wait, not gait again. We already have that concern with PD (shuffling), and it's also a concern with muscle strength loss?" And here is where the double whammy I mentioned earlier comes into play—losing muscle strength can lead to frailty.

Dynapenia, Like Sarcopenia, Is Preventable, Through Strength Training

When dynapenia sets in people walk slowly and are unstable. They eventually become frail and experience fatigue when trying to accomplish everyday activities, and they are prone to falls and fractures. Sadly, they often end up using a cane, a walker, or even a wheelchair. However, unlike PD, this situation is entirely preventable. "With identification of sarcopenia and dynapenia in the early stage among patients with IPD [Idiopathic Parkinson's Disease] diagnosis, it will be possible to continue to improvement of clinical results of the disease using precautions such as administering protein supplementation in diet to improve muscle functions and practicing resistance" (Yazar et al. 1420).

"Twenty-four percent (24%) of adults aged 65 years and older use mobility aids (e.g., canes, walkers, wheelchairs), with use increasing with advancing age. Mobility aids may compensate for decrements in balance, strength, coordination, sensation, reaction, and increased risk for falls. Falling presents a prevalent event in aging as 35–40% of community-dwelling adults age 65 years and older fall each year. As fall prevention efforts have increased, so has the use of mobility aids, which have increased by 26, 57, and 65% for canes, walkers, and wheelchairs, respectively, among all ages" (Fragala et al. 2032).

Sarcopenia Related to Age while Dynapenia is Not

In an original study titled *Sarcopenia and Dynapenia in Patients with Parkinsonism* (Barichella et al. 2016), the objective was to "estimate the prevalence of sarcopenia and dynapenia in outpatients with PD and to investigate their association with the features of the disease" (Barichella et al. 640). A total of 235 Parkinson's disease patients participated in a study. (In total, 235 patients or (64.6%) had a diagnosis of idiopathic PD . . . while 152 patients actually had PD.) "Low SMM [skeletal muscle mass] index was recorded in 27 patients . . . Prevalence of sarcopenia and dynapenia was 6.6% (95% confidence interval [CI] 4.3e9.7) and 75.5% (95% CI 70.8e79.9), respectively" (Barichella et al. 640).

Sarcopenia is mainly related to advancing disease, which is not the case with dynapenia. "Dynapenia was more frequent in women (P ¼ .021) and non-PD parkinsonism (P ¼ .003) and unrelated (P ¼ .793) to the ability to perform GS [gait speed] assessment, disease duration, and severity. It was directly associated with older age, smaller calf circumference, and disability, whereas physical therapy appeared to be a preventive factor. Patients with dynapenia had also lower GS" (Barichella et al. 643).

All Aboard the PD Resistance Exercise Train, Tickets Are Selling Like Hotcakes

After reading this next section you should be more than ready to buy a train ticket to progressive strength training, the most effective intervention to prevent, slow down, and treat sarcopenia and dynapenia. Strength interventions can minimize the destructive effects of immobility, manage chronic disease, and

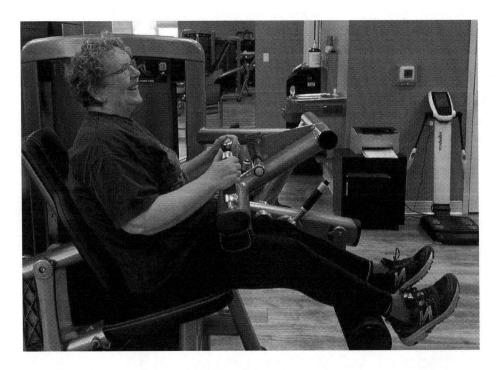

Kay Arvidson found out that resistance training brought a whole new level of freedom and empowerment to her battle against PD. Here she is working to strengthen her legs on the leg curl machine.

improve physical functioning, psychological well-being, and quality of life. "Current research has demonstrated that countering muscle disuse through resistance training is a powerful intervention to combat muscle strength loss, muscle mass loss (sarcopenia), physiological vulnerability (frailty), and their debilitating consequences on physical functioning, mobility, independence, chronic disease management, psychological well-being, and quality of life" (Fragala et al. 2019).

NSCA Warns of Debilitating Consequences if Older Adults Don't Strength Train

The National Strength and Conditioning Association (NSCA) released its position on resistance training for older adults in October 2019 (Fragala 2019-2052). The Position Statement detailed that an older adult's exercise program should include a combination of strength, power, and endurance to counteract declines in muscular strength, mass, cardiorespiratory fitness, neuromuscular function, and functional capacity. A 2012 review on dynapenia found that "the clinical consequences of dynapenia are significant, because it increases the risk for functional limitations, disability, and mortality" (Clark 9).

The NSCA statement includes eleven summary statements for practical resistance training regarding older adults, including people who have other neurological diseases, as well as those who are living in nursing homes. The NSCA aims to break down the fear and barriers that older adults have when it comes to resistance training. According to Rear Admiral Paul Reed, MD, Director of the Office of Disease Prevention and Health Promotion, "Only 27.6 percent of men and 20.8 percent of women in the U.S. report sufficient activity to meet the relevant aerobic and muscle-strengthening guidelines in the Physical Activity Guidelines for Americans. The latest iteration of the Guidelines cites related impacts—in dollars and deaths—indicating 'about $117 billion in annual health care costs and about ten percent of premature mortality are associated with inadequate physical activity, alone.'" (Reed "Health"). It's vital to help everyone, with or without PD, understand why exercise and strength training are essential to their quality of life as they age.

PWPD Are at Two Times Higher Risk Factor for Hip Fractures

Startling statistics put this topic into sharp perspective. A research team used the National Health Insurance Service-National Sample Cohort data collection in Korea to look at the risk of hip fractures and their effect on mortality in patients with PD in Korea. "In total, 26,570 individuals were enrolled in the study: 2,657 in the PD cohort and 23,913 in the matched comparison cohort. The PD group had about a two times higher risk of hip fracture than the comparison group . . . Regarding post-fracture mortality in patients with PD, the mortality risk was twice as high in the patients with hip fracture than in those without" (Nam et al. 544).

Progressive Resistance Exercise Research for PWPD Proves to Be Essential for Motor and Non-Motor Symptoms

A Two-Year Randomized Controlled Trial of Progressive Resistance Exercise Training for PD (later called the PRET-Study) (Corcos et al. 2013) was held at the University of Illinois at Chicago. Professor Daniel M. Corcos conducted the trial from September 2007 to July 2011; he had previously worked on research studies showing that PWPD are inherently weak, particularly during the "off" period of medication. "Patients with Parkinson's disease are slow and weak, and progressive resistance exercise (PRE) improves muscle strength, gait initiation, and gait speed. PRE in combination with other exercise modalities improves strength, decreases postural sway and decreases falls, improves whole body bradykinesia, and improves quality of life. A combination of exercise modalities including resistance, aerobic, and balance and stretching exercises is most likely to be optimal for patients with Parkinson's disease" (Corcos et al. "Two-Year" 2).

The PRE study was the first time that strength training and its effects on PD motor symptoms were studied in a controlled trial. The research objective was to look at and compare the outcomes of PWPD at 6, 12, 18, and 24 months of performing progressive resistance training versus a group that performed a stretching, balance, and strengthening exercise program (without progressive resistance weight overload over time).

The Key Point Is That the mFC Group Did Not Slowly Increase Weights Over Time, while the PRE Group Did

Two groups were formed in the trial, and the participants were tested while on and off PD medication, and they did exercise while on PD medication. "We chose mFC [Modification Fitness Counts] because it is an exercise program recommended by the National Parkinson Foundation . . . We chose the PRE program to

Chapter 9

determine if PRE not only increases strength but also reduces the signs of Parkinson's disease. The programs were identical in all aspects (duration of exercise, number of exercise sessions, and time with the personal trainer) except for the specific exercises. Patients participated in their respective interventions twice a week for 24 months" (Corcos et al. "Two-Year" 3).

The biggest difference between the two groups was that the mFC Group did not progressively increase the weight load over time with the strength-training portion of the program. The mFC mostly consisted of stretches, balance, and non-progressive strengthening exercises (Corcos et al. "Two-Year" 3–4).

Progressive Resistance Exercise Doesn't Pull Punches and Puts PWPD on a True Strength-Training Regimen

The PRE Group, on the other hand, was a true strength-training program with classic weight-training exercises. It consisted of eleven strengthening exercises that progressively increased the load of the weights over time. The research stated, "At the first visit with the personal trainer, a one-repetition maximum (1RM)—the maximum amount of weight the subject can lift for one repetition—was established for each exercise. Resistance was set at approximately 30%–40% of the 1RM for upper body exercises and 50%–60% of 1RM for lower body exercises during the first week of training (Corcos et al. "Two-Year suppl" 2).

The research team went on to say, "As soon as the subject was able to perform a set of exercises using good form and perceive the exercise to be somewhat easy, the resistance was increased." The participants for both programs worked out two times a week with a personal trainer to ensure exercises were performed safely and with correct form and were evaluated at 6, 12, 18, and 24 months of exercise (Corcos et al. "Two-Year suppl" 1).

Research Results Show That Strength Training for Two Years Significantly Improves the Motor Symptoms of PD

It's not surprising that the PRE Group was the one that got impressive results. The severity of motor symptoms was measured using the UPDRS after 24 months of exercise. "We think that PRE was more effective at reducing the UPDRS-III score and improving strength for five reasons. First, the resistance used is much greater in PRE . . . Second, PRE progressively increases the resistance over time, whereas the mFC is a non-progressive training program . . . A third reason why PRE might be more therapeutic than mFC is that repetitively generating large forces increases neuronal activation in basal ganglia circuits more so than small forces . . . Fourth, reduced corticomotor excitability with force generation has been demonstrated in patients with Parkinson's disease using transcranial magnetic stimulation . . . Finally, in terms of motivation, PRE was designed to continuously challenge the patients, and they may have found this rewarding and motivating" (Corcos et al. "Two-Year" 6-7).

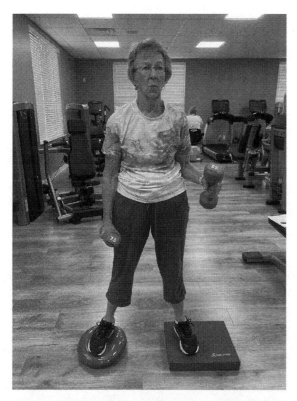

Linda O'Hair is demonstrating RTI. She is doing bicep curls with one foot on a balance pad and the other on a balance disc. Like every other kind of training, you work your way up slowly when adding a higher level of balance difficulty. Make sure you feel absolutely comfortable before the next challenge.

Resistance Training With Instability (RTI) Improves Mobility, Motor Signs, Cognitive Impairment, and Quality of Life in Patients With PD

If you aren't ready to hop on the PD resistance workout train yet, this should make you line up to buy a ticket. A 2016 Brazilian research study titled Resistance Training with Instability for Patients (Silva Batista et al. 1678–87), found that adding a bit of instability (a foam pad or a BOSU balance-training device) to your training brings a whole new level of benefit to your workout. "There is evidence suggesting that exercises requiring a high degree of attention, memory, and motor difficulty (i.e., high motor complexity) produce higher cortical activation than low motor complexity exercises. Increases in exercise-induced cortical activation are related to improvements in motor control and cognitive function in healthy individuals. Thus, exercise interventions with high motor complexity may help alleviate deficits in mobility, motor signs, and cognitive impairment of patients with PD" (Silva Batista et al. 1679).

So now you have training that improves motor, non-motor, and cognitive function. What does resistance training with instability (RTI) mean? It's simply means adding a relatively unstable device like a balance pad, disc, BOSU, or Swiss ball to the workout while you squat, perform a bicep curl, or do some other exercise while standing on the device. This kind of workout requires many things to happen at the same time. You must focus, use your muscles as the load increases, and maintain stability simultaneously. "It has been suggested that mobility impairment (postural instability and gait difficulty) is the main determinant of poor quality of life and disability, and is a predictor of reduced survival in patients with PD. However, mobility impairment represents a therapeutic challenge because pharmacological treatment (dopaminergic medication) has limited effects" (Silva Batista et al. 1678).

The Brazilian study had three groups. Group C, the control group, did no weight training. The resistance training (RT) Group only did progressive resistance training, while the resistance training with instability (RTI) group performed progressive resistance training with different balance challenges. The types of progressive resistance exercises both non-control groups used were like the ones we talked about in the previous progressive resistance exercise study.

Both RT and RTI were performed in a gym for 50 minutes twice a week for three months (24 training sessions), during which the training load progressed from high-volume repetitions, low-intensity to low-volume repetitions, high-intensity loads over twelve weeks. "For the RT group, the load/resistance of the exercises was progressively increased throughout the intervention whenever patients were able to perform two consecutive sessions with the same exercise load. For the RTI group, there was a progressive and concomitant increase in load/resistance and degree of instability of the exercises during the three months. Unstable devices were changed throughout the experimental period from the least to the most unstable devices" (Silva Batista et al. 1680).

Instability During Progressive Weight Training Adds a New Dimension to Brainwork and Imposes High Demand on the Central Nervous System

As expected, both non-control groups improved in strength, balance, and movement. These are all measures Professor Corcos' PRE study previously showed. However, the new RTI study showed some benefits in a shorter time. The results showed that over the twelve-week period, "[. . .] only RTI was effective in improving mobility, motor signs, cognitive impairment, and quality of life in patients with PD, whereas both training regimens were equally effective in improving muscle strength. Thus, exercise interventions aiming at improving mobility of patients with PD should include investigation into not only interventions that prioritize increase in muscle strength, but also mainly exercise interventions while imposing high demands to the CNS [central nervous system] in patients with PD. Therefore, this randomized controlled trial describes an innovative intervention able to counteract some PD-related effects" (Silva Batista et al. 1686).

American College of Sports Medicine's FITT PD Resistance Training Recommendations

The FITT (Frequency, Intensity, Time, Type) recommendations for individuals with PD resistance workouts are as follows:

- **Frequency:** 2–3 days a week
- **Intensity:** 30%–60% one repetition maximum (1RM) for individuals beginning to improves strength; 60%–80% 1RM for all advanced exercisers
- **Time:** 1–3 sets, 8–12 repetitions, beginning with 1 set and working up to 3 sets
- **Type:** For safety, avoid free weights for individuals in more advanced stages of the disease; focus on weight machines and other resistance devices (e.g., bands, body weight) (American "ACSM Guidelines").

Progressive Resistance Exercise Training for PWPD

The information provided regarding progressive resistance exercise training for PWPD comes from Dr. Daniel Corcos' *A Two-Year Randomized Controlled Trial of Progressive Resistance Exercise for Parkinson's Disease* Supplemental Material (Corcos et al. "Two-Year suppl" 2013). For safety reasons, PWPD should work one-on-one with a certified personal trainer who has the experience and credentials to work with PWPD (see Chapter 11).

Meeting With Your Certified Personal Trainer to Guide You through Progressive Resistance Training

When you meet with your Certified Personal Trainer (CPT) for the first visit, they will do strength tests to determine your muscular fitness. They want to see if you have muscle imbalance and determine how they will track your progress. They will perform the 1RM test (initially at 30%–60% of maximum weight) as a baseline measurement to set your strength-based goals. Your goals, abilities, and current fitness level will all come into play in determining how to approach the workout safely. The trainer will use a percentage of the 1RM weight to calculate how much weight you will be lifting for each weight exercise from that point on. For example, say you can lift 75 lbs. on the chest press machine for your 1RM. Then, the CPT will determine how many reps you can do by calculating 60% of the 75 lbs. The CPT will then have you attempt 12 repetitions at 45 pounds.

What to Expect From a Progressive Resistance Training Session

Once the CPT has determined the appropriate weight, the first session will begin. First, your trainer will have you perform five-to-ten minutes of cardio to get the muscles primed for what's coming next. Second, you'll do a few dynamic stretches to keep warming up those muscles—movements like arm circles, hip circles, or trunk rotations. Then comes the actual strength workout, which may include some of the following exercises:

1. The chest-press machine
2. The lat pull-down machine
3. The leg-press machine
4. The seated bicep-curl machine
5. The shoulder-press machine
6. The seated triceps extension
7. The leg-extension machine
8. The rotary calf machine

Exercise machines are considered safer for PWPD because you are sitting in a machine, so there is no fall risk. However, your CPT may also have you incorporate free weights (dumbbells, barbells, and kettlebells). Free weights create a balance challenge because they require you to stabilize and balance your body weight. Stabilizing your body weight while performing a weighted exercise fires the primary muscle groups you're targeting in your workout as well as all the stabilizing muscles. You will build strength regardless of which type of weights you work with—that is, if you train at least twice a week. Your CPT will work with your physical therapist or exercise professional to build a long-term program for your PD exercise journey.

Strength Training Case Studies
DawnElla M. Rust (Nacogdoches, Texas; Salida, Colorado)

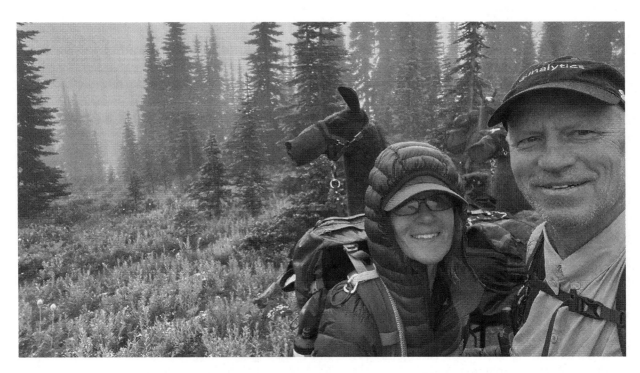

DawnElla Rust, left, and her husband, Rusty, hiked 35 miles on the Pacific Crest Trail in the Cascade Mountains of Washington State in conjunction with Pass to Pass, an organization that provides multi-day trips for people with PD (PasstoPass.org). They also have the cutest llamas for support.

"Live Life to the Fullest Despite PD" Is DawnElla's Mantra

DawnElla Rust never gives up. Whether she is hiking a mountain, helping her students, meeting her friend to work out, or kicking PD's ass every day—"defeat" is not in her vocabulary. She isn't wired to surrender. As an athlete in her youth, she learned firsthand how to push her mind and body when she didn't think she could anymore. She was diagnosed with PD in 1990 at the age of 47, but for the past thirteen years, she has lived life to the fullest. She is a full-time science health professor at a university, and in the 2018–2019 academic year was recognized with the highest honor the university bestows upon a faculty member: the Regents Scholar. She isn't letting PD define her. Instead, she is defining her life.

Exercise Is the Answer When You Are Having a Bad PD Day

That isn't to say that DawnElla doesn't have bad PD days. When I pulled her up on the Zoom screen to interview her and asked her how she was doing, she said, "I'm having one of those bad PD days," to which I replied, "Oh, we don't like those bad PD days." She responded, "You know, we don't, so as soon as we get done, I'm going to find my exercise buddy. Yes, that will definitely help." And I agreed with her that from my perspective as an exercise coach, her strategy is the best anyone with PD can have. We discussed how sometimes it might seem easier to go home and not do anything on a bad PD day. However, DawnElla shared from her experience that she feels worse if she does that. She only feels better if she works out and "clears the PD cobwebs."

Exercise Has Been and Will Always Be a Big Part of DawnElla's Life

DawnElla knows a lot about exercise. In addition to being a long-time athlete, her undergraduate and master's degrees are in health and physical education. She holds a doctorate in health promotion, and she is a professor of health science. She was in tune with her body when her physicality started going off the rails, and she went to a movement disorder specialist, who diagnosed her with PD and put her on PD meds. However, for her, exercise is the key. It has always been the answer to challenges in her life, and PD isn't any different.

Grab Those Kettlebells, A Friend, and Get Ready to Work

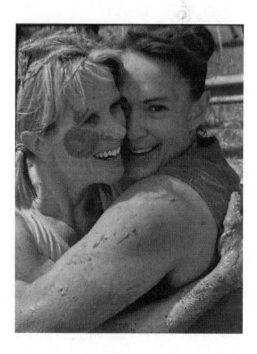

Dawn-Ella's friend, Loree McCary, became her exercise buddy. For twenty years, they have been working out together. Loree doesn't have PD, but that doesn't matter—they hold each other accountable and don't let each other slack off. Loree will ask DawnElla, "Are we doing two or three rounds?" DawnElla laughs, "I don't know why she always asks this. We always do max rounds."

I have to say that I would be huffing and puffing with one of their workouts, which aren't for the faint of heart. DawnElla showed me a PowerPoint of their exercise plans. They use sizeable kettlebells for strength workouts, along with jumping jacks, squats, bench presses, pull-ups, and of course, everyone's favorite, burpees. They even run up the football stadium ramp. We are talking 50-and 60-year-old women! I salute them both.

DawnElla Rust (left) and her exercise buddy, Loree McCary, keep each other accountable. Loree doesn't have PD, but she doesn't let DawnElla off easy just because DawnElla does.

They work out Mondays and Wednesdays, with DawnElla choosing Monday's workout and Loree choosing Wednesday's. But watch out for Saturday, because Saturdays are a group day when everyone is invited. Many have joined, but not many return—except their husbands, as they try to hang with the ol' girls.

As the Song From Madagascar Goes, "She Likes to Move It, Move It, Move It!"

Along with strength training, DawnElla likes to cycle and hike. She, her husband Rusty, and a group with PD hiked thirty-five miles on the Pacific Crest Trail in the Cascade Mountains of Washington State in conjunction with Pass to Pass, an organization that provides multi-day trips for people with PD (PasstoPass.org). They also have the cutest llamas for support.

DawnElla shared, "I love to hike. I've always been one of those people who finds ways to move. I think some people avoid moving, and others find ways to move. I've always been a mover. And my husband can tell if I haven't moved on a particular day, and he'll say, 'I can tell you haven't moved today. So go out and move because you're not very happy.'"

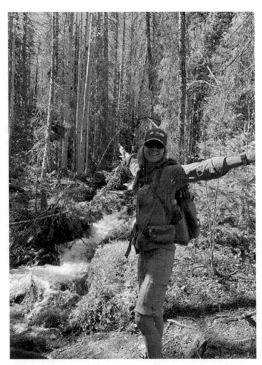

DawnElla's mantra is to "Live Life to the Fullest" despite PD. She is able to do so through exercise. It has been her "secret weapon" for the last 13 years.

Embrace Movement from Day One of Your PD Journey

DawnElla finds that her workouts help with her symptoms and her brain—which is essential, since she's a full-time college professor. When I asked her how her students viewed her, she said that she had been described as follows: "'Dr. Rust is most remarkable because she genuinely cares for her students and has a grateful outlook on life.'"

I then asked her to share what she would tell a group of newly diagnosed PWPD. She said, "I would say to them to embrace moving from day one. And to do more today than you did yesterday. And I think it's important to keep finding different ways you like to move throughout your life. Also, make sure you move with a friend or a mentor. Lastly, if you don't move, PD wins."

Strength Training Case Studies
Trent MacLean (Santa Monica, California)

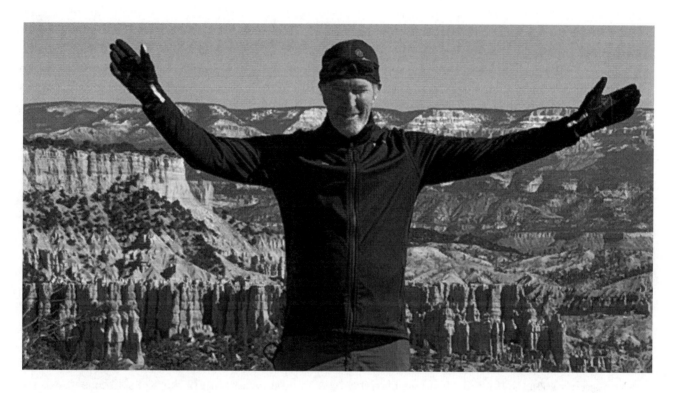

Trent MacLean has found that consistent exercise enables him to go on adventures like hiking in Utah.

From Worried Kid to Cool-as-a-Cucumber Guy With PD

"I was worried all the time as a kid," explains Trent MacLean, who grew up in Canada. "I had every disease under the sun. I grew up with asthma, eczema, food allergies, edema, temporomandibular joint dysfunction, and several concussions. And trust me, the list goes on." As a result, Trent wasn't alarmed when he started having strange symptoms at age 18. His childhood medical battleground made him impervious to anything alarming in adulthood. There were times Trent couldn't grip the tennis racket with his right hand, and his right big toe felt funny so he didn't have control skiing sometimes. These symptoms didn't worry him. They went as fast as they came, so it didn't seem like a big deal. Over the years, when these symptoms did reappear, two medical theories were that he had inflammation of his nerve endings or side effects from a nasty flu in his youth.

He Knew Something Was Wrong and was Waiting for the Other Shoe to Drop

However, thoughts still stuck in the back of his mind. He didn't believe his symptoms were nerve endings. For decades, he mulled over three possible diseases: multiple sclerosis (MS), amyotrophic lateral sclerosis (ALS, which is often called Lou Gehrig's disease), or PD. Time passed, and his symptoms kept coming and going until one day, he was cycling in the Santa Monica Mountains when he realized his symptoms had gotten far worse. As Trent was climbing a hill he had cycled many times before, he brought his foot around to complete the pedal stroke . . . and he couldn't. He said, "For me not to be able to finish on a hill that I've done routinely for years was the final sign I had been waiting for all those years. I knew it was time to face what was taking hold in my body."

He Was Relieved when They Told Him It Was PD

So, off Trent went to a neurologist in Beverly Hills. He anxiously waited for the bad news. When the neurologist proclaimed, "You've had an event!" Trent looked at him dumbfounded and said, "What does that mean?" The neurologist said, "Well, you know, you're a young guy [he was 55 at the time]. So, go to the gym and work out and you'll be fine." And with that, the doctor sent him on his way.

Trent told his friend, a semi-retired neurologist at the University of California, Los Angeles, what had happened. His friend thought otherwise about the diagnosis. He sent Trent to UCLA to do the same tests, and that neurologist reached a different conclusion. The neurologist said, "I'm 95% sure what this is, but we will do another test for confirmation." So, the doctor from UCLA sent Trent home with medication; if his symptoms improved within two days of taking the medicine, this would confirm the diagnosis. Trent improved in two days. He said, "I was grateful the day I got diagnosed with Parkinson's disease. It was such a relief. Wow. I was thrilled on that day for two reasons. One, I knew for thirty-seven years that something was wrong with my body. And two, of the three diseases I thought I had, I got the one I would have chosen."

Strength Training From a Very Young Age Was a Good Thing

Although Trent was often sick in his youth, that didn't stop him from playing. He and his brother played on high-level competitive teams—box lacrosse (an indoor version of lacrosse) and football. His love of weight training began in high school with the help of Arnold Schwarzenegger and *Muscle & Fitness* magazines. Trent laughed, "I bought all the magazines and made myself an expert to my fellow football-playing buddies back then." He built a gym in the basement, including squat racks of old wooden Coke cases, and developed a weight training program for the team. He then coached the offensive backfield players three times a week down in the basement. He continued his strength training endeavors throughout his life.

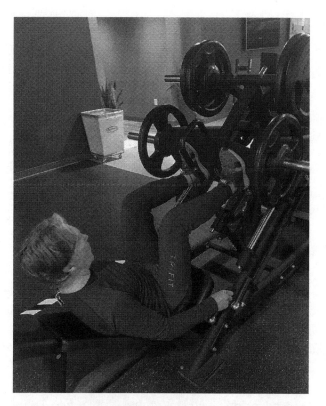

Trent's strength training equipment has been upgraded from the old wooden Coke cases from his youth. Today he advocates progressive strength training to others to help control PD symptoms.

Trent Believes His Lifetime Intense Active Lifestyle Kept His Disease in Check

Sports was Trent's family's lifestyle. It was helpful because although they moved quite a bit over the years, participation in sports always made resettling easier. His father was a hockey goalie for the Canadian Navy, and his mother was a softball player for the Canadian Navy. "I attribute my cumulative intense athletic lifestyle to the slowing of the progression of my disease," said Trent. "And on my last visit with my neurologist, I received a reduction in one of my medications because I didn't seem to need it due to my exercise program. And a thirty percent reduction in dosage is significant."

Trent is a big believer in the power of exercise for PD. He strength trains and attends indoor cycling classes and also bikes outdoors. He understands the power of exercise on his disease: "Imagine you have something that someone tells you is progressive, and you're aging. So, both of those things are working against you. However, you find out exercise has been proven to help with PD symptoms, can help with slowing pro-gression, and is natural. On top of that, exercise can help reduce medication. So, why wouldn't you exercise? Isn't this excellent news? To get better as you're supposed to be getting older and having a progressive disease? It's incredible."

Strength Training Gives Him Confidence in His Body, Particularly When It Comes to Balance and Flexibility

Trent feels that resistance training has given him the most confidence in his body, particularly regarding balance and stability. "When I hike or come quickly downhill," he said, "it's almost like mogul skiing, where you plant one foot, and you plan where the next foot goes. My confidence is so high when I know I can rely on making that plant with my foot and I have the leg strength to make it stick. So, it's my insurance policy for potential disruptions in gait, where I know that I'm not going to fall, but if I did, I could take it. I also know how to fall safely from my martial arts. I'm not your average 67-year-old man with PD because of my attention to balance and flexibility. But without my strength resistance work, I wouldn't be confident to do half of the things I do daily. And most people I meet don't realize I have PD, and I attribute that to my well-rounded, intense exercise program."

Chapter 9

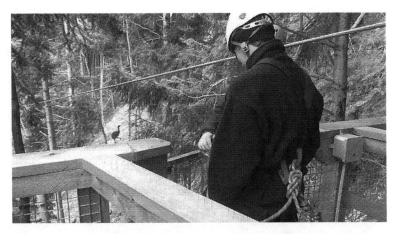

Trent MacLean likes to help other PWPD work out so they can find their way back to the things they love. Trent loves adventure and won't let PD stop him from seeing the world. Exercise lets him keep doing things like ziplining in Australia, which he is preparing to do in this picture.

Working With PWPD Is One of Trent's Passions in Life

Trent loves to work with PWPD. It is one of the things PD has changed in his life. He has met amazing people and helped change their lives for the better. For example, Trent worked with a wonderful woman in her 70s. She was previously very active but had reached a point where she just sat on the sofa without budging. She had given up on life and wouldn't even leave her condo to have lunch with "the girls" because she was afraid of falling.

"I told to her, 'You are a great skier and tennis player. Why have you given everything up?'" asked Trent.

"I can't do it anymore. I might fall, and I don't have any confidence in going out. I don't even want to try. I might have to take my walker," she said.

"So, I asked her to show me where her gym was in her condo. As we were heading to the manager's office to get a key, she had to stop five times because she was out of breath. I got the key, and we went to the gym, and it was the same stop-and-go, every few feet. I felt so bad for her. She got on the exercise bike, which took off all the tension, and I had her ride very easily for ten minutes.

"Fast forward three months later. She was almost running with her walker to the gym, choosing ten- and twelve-pound dumbbells for her weight workout. She rode twenty minutes on the bike with a resistance level of four out of ten, and her only complaint was that she was going out for lunch with the girls and didn't want them to see her with a walker. I said, 'Tell them you just had knee surgery.'"

Progressive Strength Training Is Crucial for Everyone, No Matter How Old

Trent's message to PWPD is that without a weight resistance workout routine, his friend wouldn't have had the confidence to go outside and live her life again, literally. And if you haven't done strength training before, you can start small, with no weights or a water bottle, as long as you use the proper form. "You know, you've got to fight—every day. And if it is hard, find someone to motivate you," said Trent.

Strength Training Case Studies
John Cullen (North Carolina; Seminole, Florida)

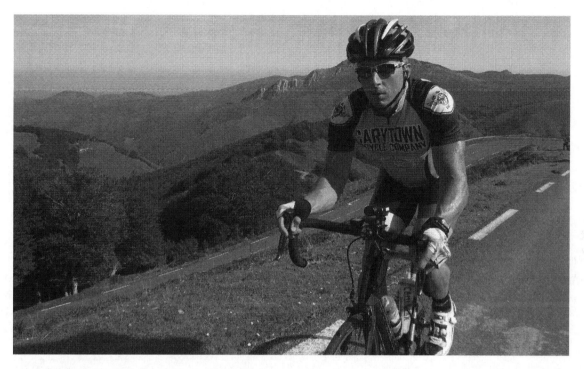

John Cullen biking up the Pyrenees Mountains in France on one of the infamous stage routes of the Tour de France.

The World Was His Oyster, until It Wasn't, and Then He Learned What Digging In Really Meant

The world was at his beck and call. Nothing ever stopped John Cullen. Life for John was about athletic challenges and pushing his body to the limit. His body always responded during the hundreds of running and cycling races and dozens of obstacle course events. That is until, he was biking up the Pyrenees Mountains in France on one of the infamous stage routes of the Tour de France—his body wasn't doing what it was supposed to do. John's right leg wasn't keeping up with the left one as he climbed up that mountain. But John wasn't going to quit. He came in dead last out of a group of thirteen riders by an hour or more every day for nine days. People, of course, wanted to know what was going on with him. Part of John wanted to know too, but part of him didn't want to know. John researched his symptoms. He narrowed it down to MS or PD. Seventeen months later, in 2015, John discovered he had PD. He was 57 years old. John's main symptoms were a weakening on the right side of his body and a slight tremor. He also experienced mental fog.

Chapter 9

If You Don't Kick It in Gear and Step It Up, PD Will Drag You Down

John wears a reminder band on his wrist that says, "Step the Fuck Up." I asked him to explain what it meant to him. He said, "To me, it means you've going to kick it in gear every day. You've got to become proactive as opposed to reactive. You must step up and work harder because PD will drag you down if you don't. And that means you gotta push for more every day regardless of where you start. It doesn't matter if you're a top athlete, you will fight harder than you ever have in the past. If you're a couch potato, you start by getting off the couch."

Initially, John didn't always apply this philosophy to himself, because he could still do most of the things he had done in the past. John thought he could take PD on and win and be the first person to beat it. But John said later that this, unfortunately, was a costly mistake because PD caught up to him quickly, and the fight was far more complicated than he had ever imagined.

On John's website, itsjustparkinsons.com, he wrote a letter to his younger self describing the issue of not hitting it hard enough in the initial stages of his PD. John says there is a sense of disbelief that you even have the disease because you feel physically okay. But that is the most crucial time to exercise the hardest before you start losing your ability to do things. He wrote to himself, "Many of your abilities will diminish (sooner than you expect or are ready for). On countless mornings, you will have trouble just getting out of bed. Your walk will suddenly become a shuffle, and you'll jokingly compare yourself to Frankenstein. Your dexterity will take a hit. Simple tasks such as buttoning and unbuttoning shirts will seem impossible. Steak knives will suddenly become unusable. Some days, getting dressed without help will be hopeless. It's okay. Ask and accept help when you need it. There is no shame. You may need assistance with certain things, but that doesn't mean you are incapable. Everyone has limitations. Be gentle with yourself. Don't allow yourself to get upset about your fate. Never blame yourself or get angry if you can't do something. Learn to roll with whatever Parkinson's dishes out. I know that's easier said than done, but a positive attitude truly is half the battle. And you, my dear John, have always been optimistic."

When He Couldn't Do the Things He Loved Anymore, He Decided It Didn't Take Much Coordination to Pick Up Heavy Stuff

John continued strength training when he could no longer ride a bike or run outside. Then one day, he saw a big guy lifting enormous weights in the gym—powerlifting. It was four years after his diagnosis, in 2019. He thought to himself, "I want to lift some heavy shit. It doesn't require much coordination. Sorry to all you powerlifters. Especially since I no longer have any coordination, and it breaks the PD stereotype—not many PD powerlifters out there. Let's do this." The big guy lifting weights ultimately became John's powerlifting coach, Vince Lamphere, Certified Personal Trainer (CPT), at Iron DNA Fitness in Florida. The goal was for John to compete in a powerlifting competition in a year and a half. It was a big challenge. John was shuffling and so rigid that his walk was almost at a snail's pace. When you watch his documentary

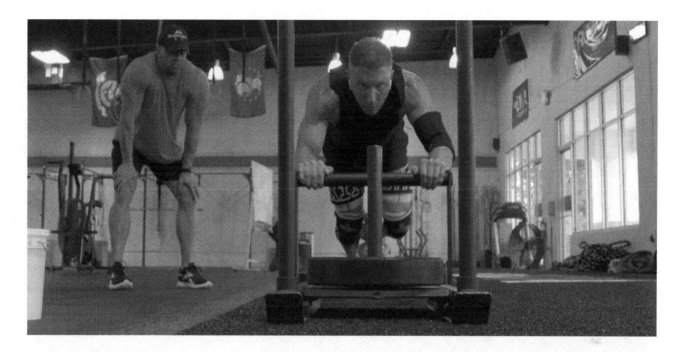

John Cullen, right, discovered that powerlifting at a high intensity relieved many of his PD symptoms. John trains with his powerlifting coach, Vince Lamphere, Certified Personal Trainer (CPT), at Iron DNA Fitness in Florida.

(vimeo.com/ondemand/itsjustparkinsons), there's a before-and-after video comparison of John walking over to pick up a loaded barbell. It shows him at the beginning of training so slow and stiff. You will be shocked at the difference six months later, walking like he doesn't have PD and picking up the barbell with ease. While training, John discovered that powerlifting at a high intensity relieved many of his PD symptoms.

Ready or Not, Competition Day Was Here Before He Knew It

After ample training, John and Vince arrived at the 2021 United States Powerlifting Association Tournament in Seminole, Florida. There was much commotion and excitement in the air. The announcer congratulated all the first-time competitors and then made a special announcement to the audience, "Up first is John Cullen, who has Parkinson's disease. I want you guys to give it up for him. I love this sport because of moments like these, it's open to anyone. He's not just coming to compete. He's coming to take some records." The crowd went crazy. They could not believe it. John walked to the squat rack. At that moment, all the noise and stimulus were too much for his PD.

John said, "It was like being in slow motion all of a sudden, and I didn't know where I was or what I was doing. I suddenly forgot how to squat." He couldn't complete his first attempt. But that didn't deter him. He went backstage and got his bearings. John talked to Vince and shook it off. He went back out there and did his second squat like it was nothing: 425 pounds. Piece of cake. The smile on his face was huge. And the crowd roared in support of him. His third squat was 450 pounds. He told the crowd, "My being here today means I don't give in to Parkinson's." And the crowd cheered even louder in support.

Chapter 9

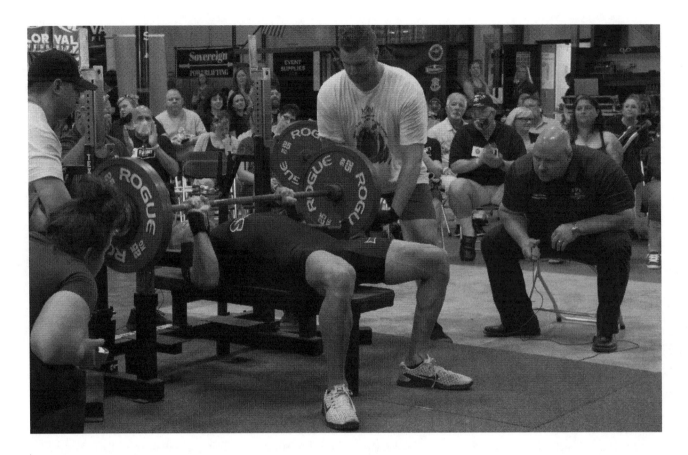

John went for a state record and just missed getting it. It was 42 pounds more than his personal record of 250 pounds. It takes courage to go to a competition, and even greater courage to go for a record 42 pounds heavier than your best press.

Not Only Did He Go to the Competition, He Attempted to Beat the State Record

John went on to attempt to break a state record on the bench press at 292 pounds, and he was inches away from getting it. His personal record before the event was 250 pounds on the bench press, which he quickly got. John also went for a personal record on the deadlift at 472 pounds but fell just under. However, he did hit his 425- and 450-pound deadlifts with ease. John went for a state record and just missed getting it. It was 42 pounds more than his personal record of 250 pounds. It takes courage to go to a competition, and even greater courage to go for a record 42 pounds heavier than your best press.

While at the event, he had many people come up and ask him about PD, and he shared his experience and knowledge. John and Vince couldn't have been prouder of how the day went. It was incredible and inspirational. John likes the motto, "No White Flags," by NFL veteran Steve Gleason, who has ALS disease. Steve says the motto means, "Resilience is the ability to transform yourself as you move through adversity or

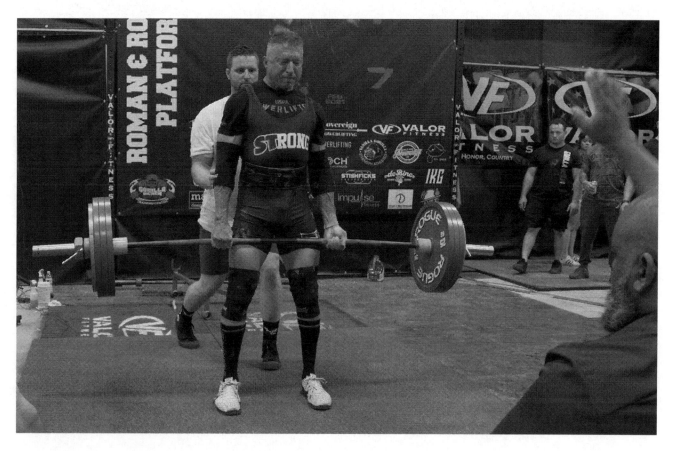

John hit his 425- and 450-pound deadlifts with ease.

painful experiences, to grow stronger, more flourishing, and more mentally free." John's journey with PD has reflected this attitude.

Remember This: I Have PD, But PD Doesn't Have Me

John would like those struggling with PD to think about the message that he wrote to his younger self and to remember it when times get tough: "Even if PD is incurable, you are still in control of your narrative. Face PD straight on and fight it with everything you have (as you have always done when obstacles have come your way). You're still the warrior you've always been. However, you now have a different shield. In time you will come to say and believe, 'I have PD, but PD doesn't have me.'"

CHAPTER 10

Parkinson's Sports Activities Exercise: Rock Steady Boxing

"Don't count the days, make the days count!"

- Muhammad Ali

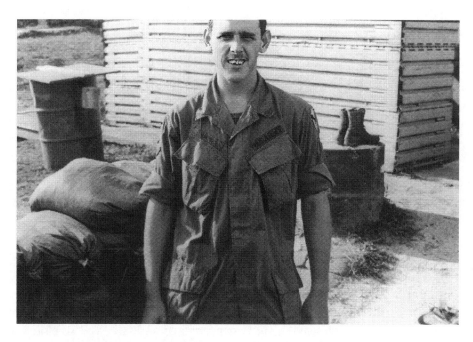

Mike Hawkins stationed in Vietnam.

More Than 110,000 Veterans Have PD Related to Agent Orange (Michael J. Fox Foundation)

Mike Hawkins didn't think he had PD when he first visited the doctor for stomach issues. However, things kept popping up, and he couldn't figure out what was happening with his body. Doctors ran numerous tests. They told him to go home after visits for random colds, viruses, and the flu. However, Mike's MRI scans concerned his family, and they set up an appointment with a neurologist, who told him she suspected PD. After more tests, Mike was diagnosed with PD.

Mike suspects he got PD from Vietnam. On June 11, 2021, the Michael J. Fox Foundation put an announcement on their website to PWPD that "U.S. Department of Veterans Affairs Expands Benefits for People with Parkinsonism Associated with Agent Orange Exposure" (Destro "U.S. Department"). Mike and other veterans were entitled to benefits from exposure to the deadly chemical while stationed in Vietnam. Mike was put on carbidopa/levodopa, and his neurologist sent him to see me for PD exercise.

Getting Set to Fight PD with a Plan of Action

Mike called me to set up a time to talk about PD exercise. We spoke on the phone for an hour about exercise and the science behind it. The last thing he said to me was, "You give me hope, and I can't wait to get started." Mike came to the facility, and we talked about the different classes and how he should start his program. Then we conducted his first assessment. At the time, Mike was a 74-year-old retired computer scientist, a little on the shy side, and not an athlete. But he understood why he needed to exercise—to help manage his PD symptoms. He was dealing with balance issues, tremors, and gait. His favorite cocktail is a Wild Turkey. His PD Exercise Cocktail Plan became Mike's "Wild Turkey—Gonna Beat You PD with a Classic!"

Ease Into Your Program at Your Pace, in Your Own Time

Mike eased into his program within a short time on the bike and a Total Health Works Total Parkinson's class. After some time, he decided he wanted to try Rock Steady Boxing (RSB), though he was hesitant at first. RSB was way out of Mike's comfort zone, but he decided to try it anyway. At first, like everyone, Mike struggled to move his body while learning the punching combinations. It's hard for many PWPD to multitask, but Mike kept going and got good at boxing and multitasking. Why? He didn't give up. Even though it was difficult for him initially, he stayed with it and found out he could do many things he didn't know were possible. He was quicker on his feet drills than he realized and had tremendous power in his punches. His stamina and endurance grew over time. Mike was quick at puzzles and games and was a great leader in team events.

In the end, Mike found out he really loved to box. He also found out that there was more to a RSB class than just boxing. He loved the camaraderie he felt in the class with his fellow boxers who have PD. He hadn't realized there was strength training, PD-specific work, other types of aerobic conditioning, brain games, theme days to celebrate holidays, and much more that happens in an RSB class. And his balance was improving; he felt more confident personally, and it showed in the way he walked and talked. RSB ended up bringing Mike joy. As the weeks and months passed, he went from being a quiet, soft-spoken person to a very talkative, happy man. He also got his cycling time up to 45 minutes. And while he started at only 60 RPM, he can now cycle easily at 80–85 RPM. Best of all, when Mike went in for his regular checkup with his neurologist, he had made significant gains in strength, gait, and balance.

Chipping Away at PD, One Day at a Time, Through Exercise

Mike works consistently and tirelessly in his quiet way. He comes daily to his classes and only misses if he has a doctor's appointment. He knows that exercise keeps his symptoms in check, and he has seen a great improvement over the last year since he began. He also enjoys the support of the group, and his anxiety and sense of isolation have greatly improved. I asked Mike what he would say to people who are sitting on the fence about trying out PD exercise. Mike said, "Everyone with PD should find a place to exercise. Try different things. I tried cycling, boxing, aqua, and brain class. It's all different and all good. It's just common sense, I think. You know, if you don't do it, bad things are going to happen. So, like the Nike ad says, 'Just Do It.'"

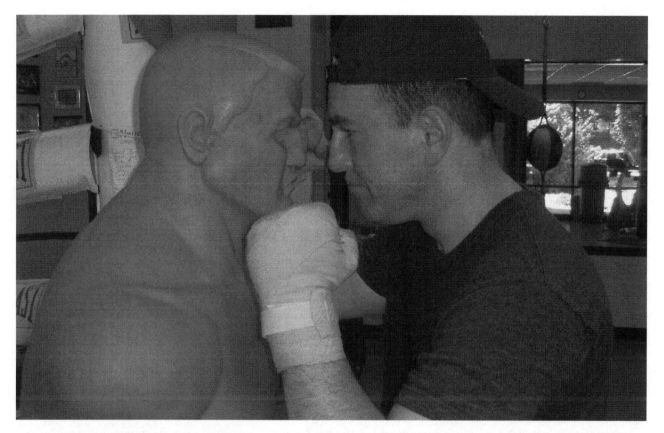

Former Marion County (Indiana) Prosecutor Scott Newman, felt mentally and physically stronger as his boxing workouts progressed.

Photo provided by Rock Steady Boxing

Former Indiana Marion County Prosecutor, Scott Newman, a PWPD, created a non-combat boxing program to help others

Rock Steady Boxing was founded by former Marion County (Indiana) Prosecutor Scott C. Newman, who is living with PD after an early-onset diagnosis at age 38. Scott is a famous politician, well-loved in the community, with a very charismatic personality. Typically, PD progresses slowly over the decades. However, Scott quickly began to lose the ability to write, talk, and walk. The disease hit Scott hard. He was trying to hide these symptoms while working, but people around him started to notice his new soft voice, shuffling feet, poor balance, tremors, and stooped posture—all classic PD symptoms.

Scott's Friend Stepped in Before PD Took Away Scott's Fight for Life

The thought of having a disease that gets worse every day for the rest of your life is daunting, depressing, and debilitating. On top of that, all of Scott's symptoms were on the fast track. The ground was sinking around him. One day, his good friend, fellow lawyer, and ex-police officer, Vince Perez (who happened to

Chapter 10

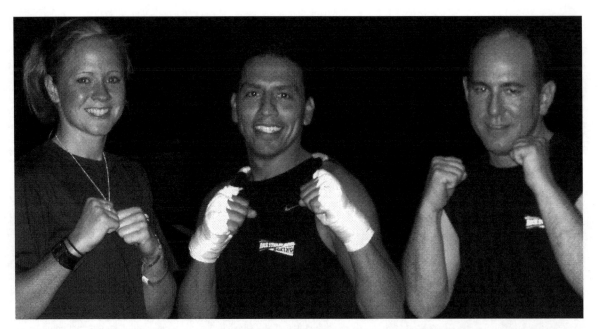

Left to right: Kristy Rose Follmar, Vince Perez, and Scott Newman founded RSB in 2006, to empower people with PD to fight back against PD. Since then, more than 50,000 PWPD have experienced the power of RSB.

Photo provided by Rock Steady Boxing

to be a former Golden Gloves Boxer), told him, "I'm not letting you go down without a fight. Let me teach you how to box because all the elements in boxing are what PD is taking away from you— strength, speed, balance, stamina, and your fight for life."

Vince took him into the ring and showed Scott the tools of the trade so he could fight back against PD. Vince worked him intensely five days a week for six weeks, and suddenly Scott was feeling better—his symptoms improved significantly. He was starting to stand up straighter, talk louder, walk better, and feel much more confident because his work in the gym was translating into results. Scott decided he could publicly announce that he had PD because he was doing something to fight it that was working. One night at dinner, Scott held out his arm (which previously had major tremors), and said, "Look, I'm rock steady." The franchise name was born.

Golden Gloves World Boxing Champion Kristy Rose Follmar Joins the RSB Co-Founder Team

Kristy Rose Follmar is a two-time Indiana Golden Gloves Women's Champion, NABC Featherweight World Champion, Super Featherweight World Champion, and WBF Light Welterweight World Champion. She said, "Scott is a brilliant man who knew if boxing worked for him, a PWPD who had rapidly deteriorating symptoms, it would be great for those on the decades timetable."

Just like Scott knew boxing would help many people with PD, he knew Kristy Rose Follmar was the perfect person to run the RSB program. He said, "It's not easy to find a caring, knowledgeable boxer to work with people who have never picked up a boxing glove, and then to change their lives."

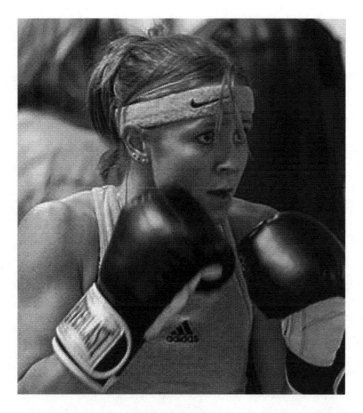

Kristy Rose Follmar is a multiple-time world-champion boxer and a 2022 Inductee into the Indiana Boxing Hall of Fame. She has helped countless PWPD and trained thousands of RSB coaches for decades.

Photo provided by Rock Steady Boxing

Being a Fighter Wasn't in Her Original Plans Growing Up

Kristy didn't know she would be a fighter growing up. Fate intervened. Her dad was a scrappy neighborhood fighter and wrestler. He taught Kristy and her brother, Thomas, to throw punches at an early age. It was something cool that they always did together. However, when Kristy was thirteen, her dad committed suicide. She was so angry she wanted to punch holes in a few doors, and she did. Her mom bought her a heavy bag and a set of boxing gloves. Kristy remembers, "My mom said, 'Go out and hit the bag when you get upset.' And that's what I did. It was so therapeutic. Back then, there weren't many boxing programs, especially for kids."

Working with PWPD Changed Kristy's Life in the Best Way Possible

Kristy heard of a program that was training kids to fight in the Golden Gloves, a program of amateur boxing tournaments. Kristy entered that gym, started fighting for real, and began a unique and unexpected career. She said, "It was always more than just the fight for me. It was very emotional because I had that connection to my dad. However, I always had a thought in the back of my mind throughout my career that I wanted to do something special after boxing, not train professional fighters. I thought it would be working with kids or boxing therapy. But, working with PWPD changed my life in the best way possible, forever."

The Rock Steady Program Is Developed and Born

At that time, there were no PD certification programs for exercise professionals. However, Kristy became a Certified Personal Trainer through the American College of Sports Medicine (ACSM) and later a Corrective Exercise Specialist through the National Academy of Sports Medicine (NASM) to allow her incredible boxing experience to safely translate into working with PWPD. Kristy is a firecracker head coach who has inspired and lifted up thousands of PWPD over the last fifteen years. She is an inspiration to hundreds of RSB coaches who have followed in her footsteps. As she often says, "Be the first responders to the thousands of PWPD whose lives are in your hands."

Chapter 10

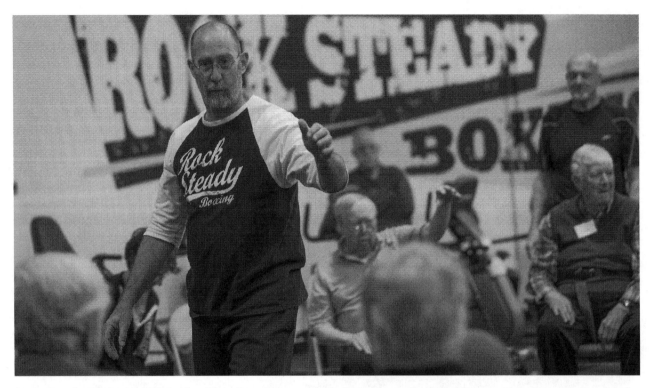

Rock Steady Boxing (RSB) can be done at any stage of PD. Classes are designed for people who use wheelchairs, walkers, and canes. Anyone can do a RSB class and get a great workout. The people in the photo are all working out from their chairs.

Photo provided by Rock Steady Boxing

First RSB Gym Opens to Small Group of Early-Onset Pioneers

In 2006, Scott, Kristy, and Vince opened a small, borrowed gym on the east side of Indianapolis, funded by private donations. They invited six young-onset PWPD to participate free of charge. The group was excited because they had seen firsthand what the training had done for Scott, and they experienced the same phenomenon that Scott had.

They improved PD symptoms and gained a better quality of life. In fact, all six original boxers with PD still train at Rock Steady Boxing Headquarters in Indiana—seventeen years later. In an interview with HBO Boxing, Scott told viewers of his own first experience with RBS: "All I know is after six weeks of intense boxing training, I was getting better. I could sign my name again. I was able to type again. I don't think I'd be sitting here today if we hadn't done this [Rock Steady Boxing]."

RSB Program Was Not What People Expected—It Was Intense Exercise, but It Was Fun and So Much More Than Boxing

The RSB program and its coaching staff grew through working with thousands of PWPD over the years. As Director of Programming and Head Coach, Kristy created a curriculum through which PWPD became

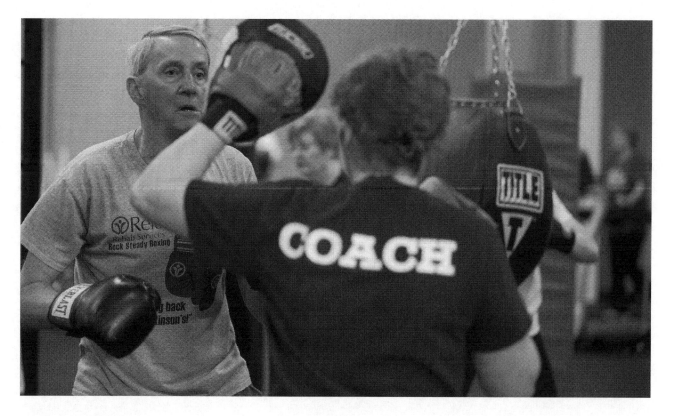

Coach Kristy Rose Follmar created a curriculum through which PWPD became stronger and more agile and improved significantly in their movement.

Photo provided by Rock Steady Boxing

stronger and more agile and improved significantly in their movement. Boxers with PD experienced life-changing results when they came to the RSB gym to work out consistently at the right intensity. At the same time, the class is fun—it has energetic music, themed events, and games that make you feel like a kid again. Not only is it uplifting for the boxers with PD, but it also helps them with non-motor symptoms like depression, fatigue, and sleep quality.

RSB Works with the University of Indianapolis Physical Therapy and Research Team

Early on, the RSB Coaching team worked with the University of Indianapolis' Physical Therapy and Research team to conduct the first studies on the RSB program. The University team followed a group of boxers with PD over a nine-month period. The 2011 article "Boxing Training for Patients With Parkinson's Disease: A Case Series" followed six PD patients who "attended 24 to 36 boxing training sessions for 12 weeks, with the option of continuing the training for an additional 24 weeks . . . The 90-minute sessions included boxing drills and traditional stretching, strengthening, and endurance exercises. Outcomes were tested at the baseline and after 12, 24, and 36 weeks of boxing sessions" (Combs et al. 132).

Chapter 10

The PWPD stayed with the program and had good results regardless of the severity of their disease. The research team found that while PWPD with milder symptoms achieved results faster, those in later stages got symptom relief as well—it just took a little longer. "Interestingly, patients with mild PD showed improvements earlier than patients with moderate to severe PD, particularly in the gait-related outcome measures. Patients with mild PD more often showed improvements that exceeded the MDC [minimal detectable change] after the initial twelve weeks of the boxing training program than did patients with moderate to severe PD. These early differences may have been due to the ability of patients with mild PD to tolerate and complete more repetitions during the circuit training regimen. This observation supports research suggesting that disease severity affects training capacity. However, patients with moderate to severe PD did eventually show improvements in most outcome measures, suggesting that they required a longer training duration to acquire the necessary training capacity" (Combs et al. 139). The Physical Therapy and Research Team and the RSB Team would go on to work together over decades, evaluating the RSB program.

The Need for RSB Affiliate Facilities Explodes

All it took was a few interviews on ABC and NBC, with boxer testimonials, and the floodgates to RSB opened wide. It seemed that everybody with PD in Indianapolis wanted to join the program. RSB staff were getting calls from people all over the country, and it was as if the world assumed there were Rock Steady Boxing affiliates everywhere. Kristy said, "It was heartbreaking. The need was so great, and we didn't have the resources yet to answer the demand."

However, thanks to being awarded the Impact 100 Health & Wellness Award for $100,000 in 2011, the organization hired its first executive director, who set up an affiliate program that established RSB facilities all over the United States. Kristy and her team created the RSB training programs and had new coaches come to RSB Headquarters in Indiana to train in the RSB method. Today Rock Steady Boxing is offered in more than 900 locations worldwide and has 43,500 participants.

Results From Combs Trial Conclusion on Rock Steady Boxing

RSB is a Parkinson's Foundation Accredited Program that provides safe and welcoming classes in local communities for PWPD to fight back against their disease. The University of Indianapolis' randomized trial noted: "This case series is the first report of the effects of boxing training in patients with PD. Provided that further reports demonstrate effectiveness, the incorporation of concepts from the whole-body boxing training regimen, such as repeated punching motions and fast-paced footwork, into traditional physical therapy treatment plans for patients with PD may be beneficial. Finding an exercise program that meets the fitness needs of a patient and that appeals to personal interests is important for long-term exercise adherence. Community-based boxing training programs for patients with PD may be a long-term alternative to physical therapy . . . the patients in this case series showed short-term and long-term improvements in balance, gait, activities of daily living, and quality of life after attending the boxing training program" (Combs et al. 140-41).

Boxers With PD Are Motivated to Keep Coming Back to RSB Because the Coaches Are Invested in Them

In a University of Indianapolis YouTube interview called *Fighting Parkinson's,* Dr. Combs-Miller commented, "For over two years of continuous boxing, [boxers with PD] were able to walk faster than people participating in other forms of exercise. We also wanted to measure quality of life. And we found over time, people that participate at Rock Steady Boxing have a higher perception of their quality of life, and they maintain that at least over a two-year period than people who do other types of exercise (Combs-Miller, "Fighting").

Dr. Combs-Miller's team also asked PWPD what attracted them to RSB, what kept them coming back, and how was RSB different from other forms of exercise. Several factors were noted including the camaraderie of the program and the fact that the participants were interacting with other people with a similar stage level of the disease that they had. They were also motivated to come to class because the coaches in the class were invested in them; there was someone there who had specialized training, understood PWPD, and cared enough about them to help them get better. The participants were also more self-motivated and wanted to improve their health (Combs-Miller, "Fighting").

A Research Study by Dr. Combs-Miller and Moore Indicated That RSB Improves Gait, Balance, and Quality of Life

In Dr. Combs-Miller and Moore's 2019 *Predictors of outcomes in exercisers with Parkinson disease: A two-year longitudinal cohort study* (Combs-Miller and Moore 2019), 88 PWPD completed testing sessions once every six months for two years (tests at baseline, 6 months, 12 months, 18 months, and 24 months). "Mode of exercise was based on each participant's self-selected exercise that they most often participated in within the six months prior to each testing session. Mode of exercise was recorded as traditional exercise (e.g., running, walking, biking, home videos, PD-specific general exercise class, or water aerobics) or non-traditional boxing exercise if the participant's primary mode of exercise was boxing or a boxing-based exercise class [Rock Steady Boxing]."

Many testing measures were used to monitor the progress of the PWPD who were part of the study. "Outcome measures across ICF [International Classification of Functioning, Disability and Health] domains of body function impairment [grip strength], activity [comfortable ten-meter walk test (10MWT)], functional reach test (FRT), activities-specific balance confidence scale (ABC), and participation [Parkinson's Disease Questionnaire-39 (PDQ-39)] were assessed at each testing session. Given the various exercise parameters expected from our sample we chose outcome measures that included upper and/or lower body movements across the ICF domains" (Combs-Miller and Moore 427).

Chapter 10

After two years, the conclusion was that the people who boxed at a higher intensity level had great improvements. "While mode of exercise varied among participants, 41 of 74 participants in the analyzed cohort reported regularly participating in non-traditional boxing training over the two years of the study. The boxing program in which all boxers in this study attended (Rock Steady Boxing, Indianapolis, IN) incorporates higher-intensity interval training with boxers encouraged to exercise as intensely as tolerated for two-to-four minute bouts as they perform various boxing activities (hitting speed bags, heavy bags, etc.) and/or different agility drills (jump rope, fast-paced foot work, etc.) followed by short, one-to-two minute rest periods. This potentially explains why those who attended boxing had a significantly higher self-perceived level of peak RPE [rate of perceived exertion] compared to all others who partook in more traditional modes of exercise. High-intensity exercise programs have shown promise in promoting short-term functional and neurophysiologic improvement in people with PD . . . Higher self-reported peak RPE during exercise predicted higher scores over time in balance self-efficacy on the ABC [a self-report measure of balance self-efficacy and confidence in performing activities in various environments] in the current study. Each one point increase on the RPE indicated an almost two point increase on the ABC" (Combs-Miller and Moore 429).

There Is a Reason Why 99% of PWPD Who Do RSB Recommend It to You

In 2019, a review paper titled High Satisfaction and Improved Quality of Life with Rock Steady Boxing: Results of a Large-Scale Survey (Larson et al. 6034-6041), was released by the Northwestern University PD and Movement Disorders Center (NUPDMDC). "A total of 2054 respondents completed the survey . . . 1709 respondents qualified for analysis. 87.7% (n = 1499) were current or previous RSB participants; 78% (n = 1333) of these were currently boxing; 210 (12.3%) respondents had heard of but never participated in RSB" (Larson et al. 6036).

"When asked 'What effect did RSB have on the following impairments?' the majority of current RSB participants reported improvement in the non-motor impairments of social life (70.3% of participants), fatigue (63.3%), fear of falling (61.9%), depression (59.9%), and anxiety (58.5%). Though not the majority, a notable proportion of current RSB participants reported improvement in select motor impairments: tremor (43.7%), falls (44.8%), freezing of gait (44.2%), and medication wearing-off (26.8%). Comparing current and previous participants' responses, there was only a statistically significant difference in percentage reporting improvement in fatigue and lightheadedness/dizziness." The paper further noted that: "Of previous participants, 90% felt that the benefits of RSB were worth the price, similar to the proportion of current participants (99%). Notably, 99% of current and 94% of previous participants would recommend RSB to others with PD." (Larson et al. 6037)

2021 Study Finds That Rock Steady Boxing Provides Value to PWPD

A small retrospective research study titled *A Community-based Boxing Program is Associated with Improved Balance in Individuals with Parkinson's Disease* found that participation in a "Community Box-

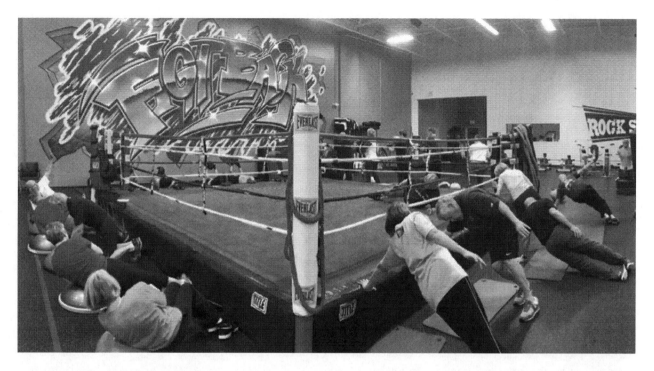

A Rock Steady Boxing (RSB) class held at RSB Headquarters in Indianapolis, Indiana, has boxers with PD performing different exercises simultaneously.

Photo provided by Rock Steady Boxing

ing Program (CBP), [Rock Steady Boxing] was associated with improved balance among clients with PD. Balance and fall risk were measured using the Fullerton Advanced Balance (FAB) Scale and the Timed Up and Go (TUG) in clients with PD . . . Sessions were 90 minutes in length involving a warm-up, boxing drills, strength and endurance exercises, and cooldown. Sessions included multiple bouts of 30-60 second high-intensity exercise intervals (RPE between 15/20 to 17/20). Results indicated a statistically significant increase and large effect in FAB performance, with a mean increase in score above previously reported minimal detectable change (MDC) . . . This study found that participation in a CBP was associated with improved balance among clients with PD." (Moore et al. 876).

The study said, "Participation in a CBP was associated with improved balance as measured by the FAB in clients with PD. Moreover, in contrast to most PD interventions that aim to slow the progression of PD by maintaining current functional abilities, participation in a CBP was associated with improved functional outcomes after attending sessions for approximately six months at three visits per week. Such findings reinforce the importance of community-based exercise programs as a valuable resource for clients navigating the challenges of chronic and progressive disease" (Moore et al. 882).

PWPD, a.k.a. Boxers with PD, Are Treated Like Athletes

RSB is a high-intensity workout, jam-packed with strength, power, balance, and endurance components, which is why it's such an effective program. The exercise is based on cardinal TRAP symptoms—tremor, rigidity, akinesia, and posture. RSB incorporates activities for the whole body. The boxing training program starts with a twenty-minute warm-up of breathing, get-to-know-ya's, chants, songs, and stretching exercises for major muscle groups. The warm-up is followed by a 45–to 60–minute circuit training regimen of functional fitness and endurance calisthenics, such as push-ups, skipping, and jumping rope, along with boxing ring work that focuses on footwork and agility drills.

RSB Has High-Intensity, Non-Combat Boxing with PD-Specific Work and Strength Training, Brain Work, and Games

The punching activities include punching heavy bags, speed bags, and focus mitts—padded mitts worn by an RSB Coach to prompt the practice of various combinations of punches toward moving targets. Boxers with PD are treated as athletes and encouraged to train as intensely as they can and to achieve more than they think is possible. The session ends with a 5–to 15–minute cooldown that emphasizes stretching, flexibility, and breathing exercises.

RSB also has special components to its workout, like fall prevention, where boxers with PD are taught how to fall in a safe manner, which helps them overcome their fear of falling, so they can participate more fully in life. Boxers with PD train to improve their balance, hand-eye coordination, speed of movement, agility, mental focus, rhythm, and muscle strength.

What to Expect When You Go to a RSB Class

In RSB, PWPD are called "boxers with PD." We like to remind our boxers with PD to remember for the next ninety minutes that they are athletes. There is a dramatic shift in the boxers' attitudes when they hear this—they feel immensely empowered. When you go to an RSB class, you will first be assessed and then assigned the appropriate class based on the results of your assessment. Your assessment will include a series of balance and movement tests.

Classes Are Divided into Levels So Boxers with PD Get the Right Training

RSB classes are divided for the boxers with PD into Levels 1, 2, 3, and 4, and classes are designed specifically for each level. A master theme, the PD focus of the week, is chosen weekly by RSB Headquarters and sent to all RSB head coaches worldwide. The theme may be bradykinesia, rigidity, endurance, speed, etc. Then it's up to the individual head coaches to create a science-based class for the boxers with PD. The head coach weaves the week's theme into all aspects of the training so that the boxers with PD are constantly working on that PD symptom theme.

This Is Not Your Average Boxing Class—It's One Where People Feel Supported, Empowered, and Like They Can Conquer Anything

RSB is much more than exercise. Time and time again, you hear boxers with PD say, "I love the camaraderie," and that is because the social connectedness felt through the class is very therapeutic. On top of

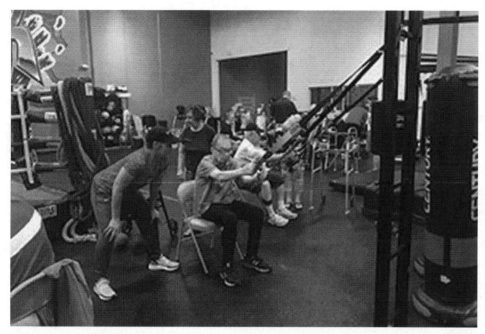

Boxers with PD perform "sit to stands" using TRX® bands at Rock Steady Boxing HQ in Indianapolis, Indiana.

Photo provided by Rock Steady Boxing

that, people experience a sense of community, acceptance, and joy. That is life-changing, because PD can be overwhelmingly isolating. For example, I once had a client come to my yearly Christmas party at our house. He was so nervous when he arrived and asked my husband, Andy, if he looked all right. My husband said that he looked great and that he was happy he could come to the party. My client then confided in Andy that it was the first time anyone had invited him anywhere in ten years. My husband wanted to cry, and I did when he told me. Connectedness is why group PD exercise is essential. The support and friendships that develop are crucial for the well-being of the PWPD.

Simply Put, PWPD Love Rock Steady Boxing

RSB is all-encompassing and uplifting. And the things you learn in a RSB class translate into functional fitness. "How does this help me in my everyday life?" And more specifically, "How does it help me with my PD symptoms?" Everything done in a RSB class is intentional and targeted to improve PD symptoms. The studies we've looked at so far have shown improvements in balance, mobility, strength, and other physical and psychological qualities that are affected by PD. The 2019 *High Satisfaction and Improved Quality of Life with Rock Steady Boxing: Results of a Large-Scale Survey* showed a 70% improvement in the current boxers' social category and a 65% improvement in previous participants (Larson et al. 6039). That reinforces that people go to RSB for the camaraderie. Simply put, they love RSB. They work hard, but have a blast while doing it.

Chapter 10

Rock Steady Boxing Case Studies
Tom and Chris Timberlake (Indianapolis, Indiana)

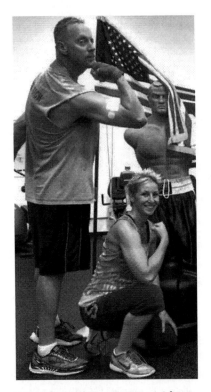

Tom Timberlake dragged his reluctant wife, Chris, to watch him during a Rock Steady Boxing (RSB) class. Halfway through, she was so excited by what she witnessed she became a volunteer. After 17 years with the program, Chris is now the RSB HQ Director of Training and Education.

In His Athletic Prime at Age 33, the Avid Athlete Couldn't Figure Out What These Strange Symptoms Were

Tom Timberlake was an avid athlete. He ran marathons and knocked the softball out of the park when he got up to bat for his team. At 33, Tom was indeed in his athletic prime. Except that he had a couple of random unexplainable symptoms happening. He felt apathetic at times—contrary to his "work out hard" mentality. His toes were curling. He asked his wife, Chris, "What the heck can that be from?" Suddenly the softball wasn't going over the fence. Hmmm. He had a sore shoulder, and Chris noticed his arms were not swinging quite as they used to when he walked. They were subtle symptoms. It wasn't even a tell-tale tremor. Chris explained, "You know at 33, why the heck would you suspect something like Parkinson's disease?"

Test after Test, Doctor Visit after Doctor Visit, Still No Answer

By 35, Tom started to display a few more motor symptoms but still no tremors. Then, years went by with visits to various doctors. Back in the 1990s, doctors weren't seeing a lot of early-onset PD patients, so many diagnoses were missed. Thus it wasn't until 1997, that Tom was finally diagnosed with early-onset PD. Chris remembers, "It was almost like the diagnosis gave the tremor permission to release. Then, the next day, his thumb started to twitch, and I was like, 'Dang, that is that is something new,' and it was like, 'Okay, PD, you're here. A guest that we didn't invite into our lives, and I guess you will not leave.' So, we were in a heap of denial because he was still functioning well—until apathy crept in, and that is definitely a symptom."

For Six Years, Apathy Took Hold and Sunk Tom Into Despair

The human reaction to a PD diagnosis is, most understandingly, despair. But on top of this, it involves the loss of dopamine, which is an important chemical in the brain that makes people happy. Tom felt all of this, plus the lack of hope. He was living in a household of athletes, but he was diagnosed at the time before PD exercise existed (it would be another nine years before a PD exercise program was developed).

Chris explained, "We were young adults. And for six years, we did absolutely nothing except for Tom taking carbidopa/levodopa. And it seemed to provide some relief. However, he became a couch potato and just got worse. All he could do was get up for work. He's six foot five. Getting him out of bed became more problematic. And getting to work at five a.m. became more stressful. So, I empathize with many young-onset folks doing their darndest to put on that face and be brave at work. You know, we call it 'the hand and pocket.' It's where you tuck the hand under the arm or in your pocket to hide the tremors at work."

Tom Lost Ground Fast, and PD Was Taking Hold at Lightning Speed

Tom tried hiding his symptoms at work. He was a tool and die maker at General Motors. There was a lot of walking and manual labor. At the time, he didn't realize how much his gait had changed. It was more of a slow shuffle. People knew he had something going on, but Tom was doing his best to hide his symptoms. By then, Tom had gotten so deconditioned, and the disease had accelerated so quickly, that he was shuffling, tripping, and choking without any exercise intervention, being only on medication.

Chris said, "I got really good at the Heimlich maneuver. Tom went downhill so fast. I think he had resigned himself to letting PD have its way. And it was because we didn't know anything different at the time. He was pretty much in the later stages of PD by then. I always cry because my heart understands this dilemma for my family and others. I know how it feels as a care partner to be unable to help the person you love get better. And I know millions of people out there are saying, 'Come on, let's do something about this,' and they don't know what to do—because they don't have the tools. So, that's what drives me today to help PWPD through RSB. I thank Tom for that. Because his story changed both of our lives."

A Small Young-Onset Group Invited Tom to the First Rock Steady Boxing Class

It was Scott Newman who got Tom out of his rapidly sinking ship. Tom had gained 40 pounds since he had stopped working out and he was also out of cardiovascular shape. He could barely get up out of a chair. Scott invited Tom to join the Young-Onset Group and attend the first-ever Rock Steady Boxing workouts, and it forever changed the participants' lives.

Despite his condition, Tom was, at heart, a competitor. That spirit was still inside him. So, he attacked the RBS workouts with a vengeance. Chris said, "Tom worked with Kristy Rose Follmar. She was tough as nails and just what he needed. So when Scott brought Kristy to RSB, it was visionary—a combination of genius, athleticism, and heart. And it rekindled a fire within Tom."

Within weeks, Tom started to stand up straighter and talk louder. And he slept better. His body was functioning and moving better during the day, which made his medications work better. His quality of life improved, and he was ready to take charge—not let PD rule. He had hope again.

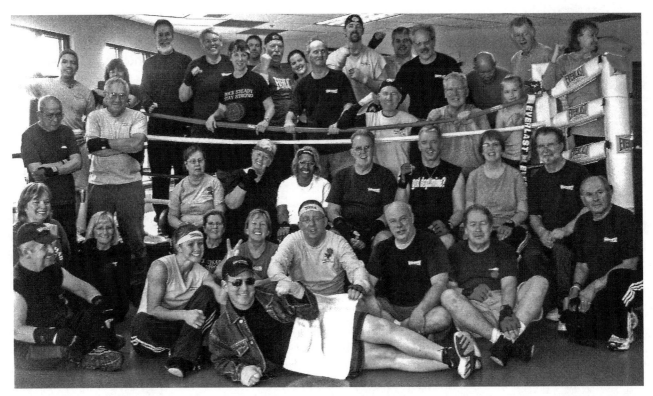

Smack dab in the middle of the back row wearing a white shirt is a smiling Tom Timberlake, posing with the original Rock Steady Boxing (RSB) crew in Indianapolis, Indiana. RBS founder Scott Newman is in front, lying down; to his left, with the headband, is co-founder Coach Kristy Rose Follmar. Tom, to this day, has the same bold attitude he had in 2003 when the photo was taken. More than 20 years into PD, he still works out at RSB HQ in Indianapolis. Most everyone in this photo is still working out today.

Photo provided by Rock Steady Boxing

Tom Was So Excited—He Couldn't Wait to Share Boxing with Chris

Tom was eager to have Chris come to class and watch the workouts. She remembered, "I told him, 'I'm gonna run; you box.' He was like 'Nah, you gotta, you gotta come!' So, I let him drag me in there. I walked in the door, and I was like, 'Oh my gosh, you guys are like rolling on the floor. Having focus mitts in your face, getting up, getting down!' The things that were happening in there. I couldn't believe it. Tom was getting up and down off the floor with no problem. I instantly fell in love with what goes on in a RSB class." And, the next thing she knew, Chris was a volunteer coach at RSB HQ.

The Same Group That Started at RSB Still Works Out There With Tom More Than Twenty Years Later

Tom, to this day, has the same bold attitude. More than twenty years into PD, he still works out at RSB HQ in Indianapolis. Chris reflects, "Wow, I'm not going to say that it's been easy, but he has his PD care team. Everyone needs to put together a PD care team. Tom has had the same neurologist for twenty-three years, a movement disorder specialist at the Center of Excellence in Indianapolis. We're fortunate to have many resources here, which I don't take for granted."

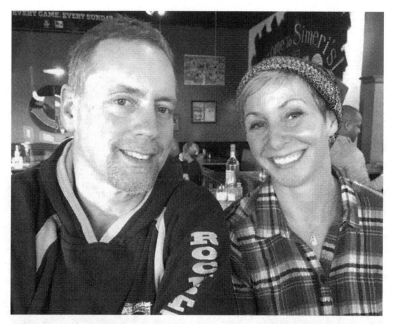

More than twenty years into PD, Tom Timberlake still works out at RSB HQ in Indianapolis. He and his wife, Chris, are fortunate to have access to a fantastic care team that includes a Movement Specialist at the Center of Excellence in Indianapolis.

Looking back over the years, Chris explain, that the most significant danger with PD is apathy. "PD operates in a sneaky way. It lulls you until you don't realize how bad the symptoms are. So, for example, if you're sitting in a chair, you probably don't know that one side of your body has stopped moving. And the other side is doing all the work. That's why a coach gets in your face and says, 'Hey, we're going to work on symmetry today. We're going to work on equal power in your punches. We're going to work on voice activation, and we're going to help you not choke.' I mean, this is an emergency. It is. It's like the house is on fire. We would have lost Tom long ago if it weren't for PD exercise and Rock Steady Boxing."

> *I mean, this is an emergency. It is. It's like the house is on fire. We would have lost Tom long ago if it weren't for PD exercise and Rock Steady Boxing.*

- Chris Timberlake, Care Partner

Chapter 10

Rock Steady Boxing Case Studies
Steve Gilbert (Indianapolis, Indiana)

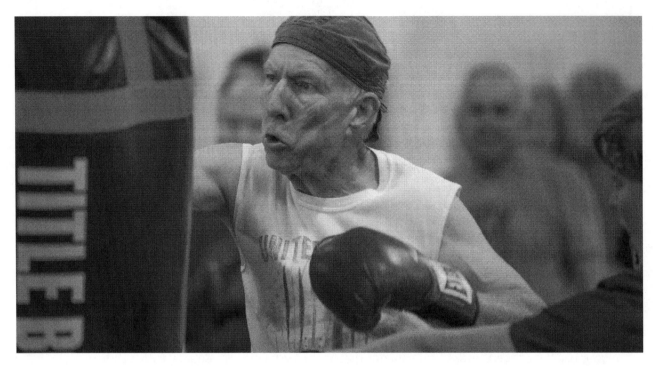

Coach Kristy Rose Follmar yells 'Come on, Steve Bean, you can do this!" Steve Gilbert was one of the early participants in the Rock Steady Boxing Headquarters class in Indianapolis, Indiana.

The Local Newspaper Ad With a Grumpy Guy Wearing Boxing Gloves Caught Steve's Eye

Sixteen years ago, an ad in the local Indiana newspaper caught Steve Gilbert's eye. The ad showed a grumpy-looking guy with boxing gloves in the first public article on Rock Steady Boxing. The story explained a new concept of non-contact boxing that was helping people with PD improve their symptoms. Steve thought, "Hmmmm, it sounds interesting." So, he got dressed and headed over to the Rock Steady Boxing gym, where a young woman with fiery red hair shouted at him, "Hello, what brings you here to the gym today?" Steve replied, "Idle curiosity."

Steve Found Out He Was Capable of So Much More Than He Realized

The first day Steve worked out there, he held back because he was the new kid. The woman with the fiery red hair was Head Coach Kristy Rose Follmar. Steve remembers Kristy yelling at him, "Come on, Steve Bean. Come over here. You can do this!" And he thought, "YES, I CAN DO IT!" Steve remembers. "Over the years, I found that I could learn to do many things I didn't think I could do. I could jump rope, hula hoop, vault horses, work with weights, and hit the speed bag. With my small band of Rock Steady brothers and sisters, three mornings a week, we got together to kick 'Parkie's' butt."

A Cancer Survivor Who Thought He Had Gotten through One Dreaded Disease to Find Out He Had to Face Another

Beyond "idle curiosity," what brought Steve to those first Rock Steady Boxing classes? His story begins in 2004. Steve had just recovered from prostate cancer surgery, and Florida was reeling from four hurricanes—Charley, Frances, Ivan, and Jeanne. In September, Steve, a FEMA contractor, was preparing to leave to do safe housing inspections when he reached for something and noticed it—the tremor. Steve went to a neurologist and was diagnosed with an essential tremor—a nervous system disorder that causes rhythmic shaking.

In November, Steve returned for more evaluations and, at 59 years old, was diagnosed with PD. Steve said, "As I stand here today and look back, I realize how blessed I was to have PD in Indianapolis because it was the only place in the country at that time that had a Rock Steady Boxing Gym. And I couldn't have done any of the miraculous things I 've accomplished without Rock Steady Boxing."

He Had Never Done Anything Athletic in His Life

Steve was never athletic as a youth or an adult. However, as he exercised at the little RSB gym, he grew physically stronger and more confident. He felt empowered and filled with a juvenile exuberance. In the spring of 2010, Steve's brother came to Indianapolis to run a half-marathon. Inspired, Steve decided to run with him. Steve said, "It was crazy to just up and decide to run a half-marathon with my brother at the last minute. I started the race not properly rested, and when I began to fatigue halfway through, I momentarily thought of dropping out. Then I quickly reminded myself that quitting is not what we do at the RSB gym. We work hard for three minutes and then take a minute off. So, I'd run for three minutes and then walk for a minute, and that's how I finished the race. I finished well behind my brother, but what was important to me was that I finished my first half-marathon." Steve used this on-and-off training strategy for the 2023 Boston Marathon, which he ran at the age of 77.

Always Good to Have the Roadies With You on Race Day

The following year, his roadies—Kristy Rose Follmar, Christine Timberlake, and her husband Tom Timberlake—cheered him on as Steve ran his marathons. In 2014, Steve began training with Matt Ebersol of Personal Best Training (PBT). The collaborative relationship between PBT and RSB enabled Steve to post his best time at five distances the year he turned 70.

Chapter 10

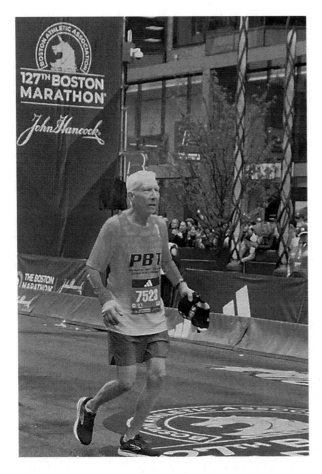

Steve Gilbert was never an athlete, but after being diagnosed with PD and training at RSB, he became a marathon runner in his seventies. Here he is, running the 2023 Boston Marathon at the age of 77.

Steve Takes Pride in Being a RSB Pioneer

When I interviewed Steve, I asked him how it felt to be a PD RSB pioneer. He answered, "I take a little pride in our little group being there from the beginning. And it grew to 16 to 24 to 38 people, and then we needed a new building. Nevertheless, the organization's growth was good—more PWPD were being helped. And look where we are today, with RSB affiliates all over the world, and there still aren't enough of them. What's most impressive is that the original core group of us that started 16 years ago are all still working out at RSB Headquarters in Indiana. Of course, we have said goodbye to a few boxers with PD along the way, but it is amazing how many are still hitting the bag. That says a lot about the program."

PD Awakened the Athlete He Never Knew Existed Inside of Him

Steve has worked out three times a week at the RSB gym in Indiana for 16 years. High-intensity exercise has enabled him to run marathons, climb 14,000-foot mountain peaks in Colorado and Wyoming, and hike the Inca Trail to Machu Picchu, a 26-mile stretch of difficult-to-hike, uneven stone pavers. ming, and hike 14,000-foot mountain peaks in Colorado and Wyoming, and hike the Inca Trail to Machu Picchu, a 26-mile stretch of difficult-to-hike, uneven stone pavers. Steve's neurologist said, "I didn't know you before PD, but I know you would not be what you are today without Rock Steady Boxing." Steve knows that to be true as well. "Rock Steady Boxing slowed the progression of my disease and kept my symptoms under control for a very long time because I was fortunate to start boxing soon after I was diagnosed," he said. "It also awakened something I had never been or thought I would be—an athlete. I thought you had to be born an athlete. Instead, I found out that it's a state of mind. Different people have different potentials, and anybody can do it. If they're committed. And I think many people need to hear that if they have PD."

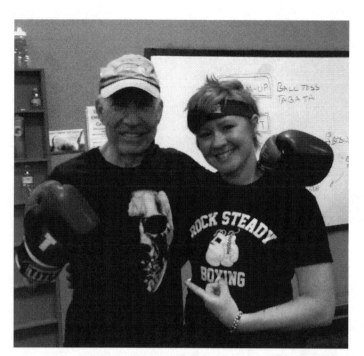

Steve "Bean" Gilbert, left, with his favorite coach, Kristy Rose Follmar. "She can inspire like no other," said Steve.

None of This Could Have Been Done Without My Cornerman, a.k.a. Care Partner

Steve's wife, Donna, was his cornerman (a boxing term that refers to a coach or trainer who assists the boxer during a bout) long before he realized she had taken on this critical role. She encouraged him to get a medical opinion on his tremor and then to make that first trip to the Rock Steady Boxing class. Donna waited in the cold through Steve's long first marathon and convinced the DJ to play the theme from "Rocky" as Steve and his brother exhaustedly approached the finish line. She took on the security guys at Steve's half-marathon when they told her she couldn't watch him cross the finish line, "My husband is 70 and has PD, and you are telling me that I can't watch him finish?" They relented. She got to watch him finish. manages the day-to-day, PD non-motor and motor symptoms that sneak in and erode the quality of life a little at a time. She is the one who reminds Steve when there are unnoticed dangers of tall ladders, icy sidewalks, and other hazards of "Parkie" [Parkinson's person] life.

> *I was fortunate to start boxing soon after I was diagnosed. It also awakened something I had never been or thought I would be—an athlete. I thought you had to be born an athlete. Instead, I found out that it's a state of mind.*
>
> - Steve Gilbert, PWPD

Chapter 10

CHAPTER 11

How to Ensure That an Exercise Professional Is Qualified to Work with PWPD and How to Find PD Exercise Programs

"My full-time job is keeping this body running."

- Jimmy Choi, Three-Time American Ninja Warrior, PWPD

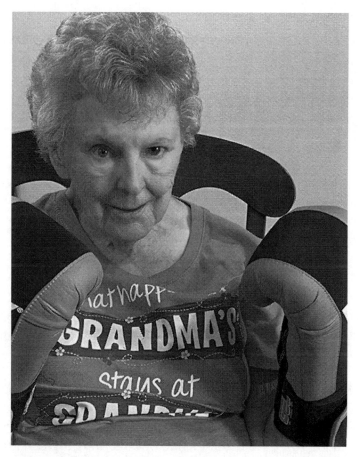

I love this photo of my client Hilda Alpin, age 79. We took it to show her grandchildren that she loves to box. Hilda works out against PD for her family. Hilda has fun in class and loves to sing and boogie to the music. Part of my job when working with my clients is to educate them on how to find qualified professionals when they are entering new programs, for their safety and well-being.

How Do I Ensure That an Exercise Professional Who Works with PWPD Is Qualified to Work With Me?

I want to talk about some essential things for you to act on the minute you leave the neurologist's office, after they've told you, hopefully, to exercise. First, as you will learn from many of the stories in this book, you need to find a physical therapist and/or certified exercise professional with the right experience and credentials working with PWPD to help you build your PD Exercise Cocktail Plan™.

You should interview anyone you are potentially going to work with—it's for your safety and well-being. Do not assume that just because someone claims to be an exercise professional that the person is qualified to teach you and has experience working with PWPD. You would be shocked to learn how many are not. Additionally, many professionals let their certifications lapse and don't keep themselves in good standing with their certifying agencies. When interviewing potential exercise professionals, ask them to provide proof of current certification and to detail the amount of experience they have working with PWPD. Ask to see their credentials (non-PD and PD) at your first meeting. Every exercise professional should have either a Group Fitness Instructor (GFI) certification or a Certified Personal Trainer (CPT) certification in addition to any PD specialty certifications (Rock Steady Boxing (RSB), PWR!Moves®, etc.). They should also have evidence of continuing education course (CEC) training—which is critical in a field where new science-based exercise techniques are continuously evolving. Qualified professionals will be more than happy to show you, their credentials. Here are the questions you should ask.

1. Are you a certified group fitness instructor or a certified personal trainer? What organization certified you? How long have you been working in this capacity?
2. Do you have any specialty certifications, additional education, or background experience?
3. What PD certifications or PD CEC courses have you taken? What other areas of PD training do you have?
4. How long have you worked with people who have Parkinson's disease?
5. What safety protocols and procedures do you have in place?
6. Are you current in your cardiopulmonary resuscitation (CPR) and automated external defibrillator (AED) training?
7. Will you send my neurologist a copy of your credentials?

Understanding the World of Exercise Professionals Before We Get to Parkinson's

Why do you need to care about the exercise professional's world? So you don't get hoodwinked, and for your own safety. Many many more uncredentialed or unaccredited exercise professionals out there want to train PWPD. Knowing what qualifications to look for is in your best interests when choosing who to work with.

Who Accredits the Accreditors?

I mentioned "certification" as a critical requirement for your chosen exercise professional, but just what does "certified" mean? Anybody can hang out a shingle saying "A1 Certification Agency." Just print up some nice documents, and for a fee, allow "professionals" to say, "Certified by A1 Certification Agency."

There are, however, standards of certification in most fields, and that includes exercise professionals. For an organization to certify an exercise professional—to be able to provide those papers that they will show you at your first meeting—that organization itself must be certified and have demonstrated that their requirements for awarding a professional certification meet the highest standards and most rigorous requirements of their profession.

The National Commission for Certifying Agencies (NCCA) is the gold standard for determining which agencies can certify professionals, including exercise professionals. Founded in cooperation with the federal government in 1977, NCCA today has certification programs that range from automotive designers to crane operators. All of the exercise programs accredited by the Parkinson's Foundation require that execcise professionals have, as a primary certification, either a GFI or CPT from an NCCA-accredited organization. You too, when selecting a GFI or CPT, want to make sure they are certified by an NCCA-accredited organization. But the standards are extremely rigorous; in the fitness world, there are only a handful of agencies that make the cut. Three top-tier NCCA-accredited agencies have passed the stringent qualifications to certify group fitness instructors and certified personal trainer.

The three agencies recognized for 2023 are:

- American Council on Exercise (ACE)
- National Academy of Sports Medicine (NASM)
- International Sports Sciences Association (ISSA)

See Appendix C for six other top-tier NCCA-accredited organizations for CPTs who passed.

If It Isn't NCCA GFI/CPT Certified, It Isn't Worth the Paper It's Printed On

Lack of understanding of the certification process is a serious problem in the fitness industry. Hundreds of so-called fitness businesses are spitting out "certifications" that aren't verified by anyone and haven't been through any sort of rigorous examination of candidates' experience or their fitness to safely and effectively train the clients that come into their businesses. Unfortunately, some wanna-be instructors and trainers like to take the easy route, rather than try to meet the stringent requirements required to pass an NCCA certification. Because who is going to tell unsuspecting clients otherwise? An American Council on Exercise article titled "What is Accreditation?" warns, "All Certifications are not created equal. Be wary! There are more than 100 providers offering certification programs that are not [NCCA] accredited at all. It's a list that contains respectable organizations, fly-by-the-night operators, and providers of overnight 'credentials'" (What "Accreditation").

Another important fact about a certification is that GFI and CPT professionals who have attained their certifications through NCCA-certified agencies must re-certify every two years to ensure they keep current with the latest advances in science and the best practices of their industry.

A Certificate Is Not a Certification

Don't get fooled when someone hands you a "certificate" and says, "I'm a certified Parkinson's Trainer." Number one, there is no such thing as an NCCA-Certified Parkinson's Trainer (or Coach, or Specialist). Number two, they are comparing apples and oranges; a certificate is not a certification.

To earn a certification, applicants must pass one or more assessments to demonstrate that they are qualified to practice as "a certified" professional. Certification also includes proctored, competency-based exams. And a certification needs to be kept in good standing by recertification. It can take six to eight months to prepare for a certification exam accredited by NCCA, such as ACE or NASM, and 35% of people don't pass on the first attempt.

Chapter 11

A certificate course, by contrast, is simply a continuing education course (CEC) with the goal of participants acquiring specific knowledge, skills, and/or competencies. The course is usually a couple of hours in length. While CECs are a necessary part of an exercise professional's training, they are not a substitute for certification. While it is useful to see what courses an exercise professional has completed, as evidenced by a certificate, what you really need to see is a document that spells out that the instructor is certified by one of the NCCA-accredited agencies listed above. Remember, a "certificate" is NOT the same as a certification.

> *All Certifications are not created equal. Be wary! There are more than 100 providers offering certification programs that are not [NCCA] accredited at all. It's a list that contains respectable organizations, fly-by-the-night operators, and providers of overnight 'credentials'.*
>
> **- The Americam Council on Exercise (ACE)**

There Is No NCCA-Approved Parkinson's Exercise Specialist Certification

When searching for a PD coach or trainer you will encounter many people with titles like PD exercise trainer, PD exercise wellness coach, and PD exercise specialist. However, those titles are misleading. According to Lisa Hoffman, Director of Education at the Parkinson's Foundation, the only correct title for someone working in the PD field is "an exercise professional who works with PWPD."

The reason for the confusing situation is that none of the NCCA-approved agencies have yet to create a Parkinson's Exercise Specialist certification or certificate. Those of us who are NCCA-accredited exercise professionals working with PWPD for the past ten to twenty years have gathered one, two, three, or more Parkinson's specialty certifications, PD certificates, and PD continuing-education coursework to build up our expertise and credibility—there is, as yet, no NCCA-accredited certification for working with PWPD.

There Is No Single Source to Find Exercise Professionals Qualified to Work with PWPD

You need to select an exercise professional to work with based on their certifications, education, and experience working with PWPD. Unfortunately, there is no single place to find those people. The U.S. Registry of Exercise Professionals is one place to find qualified exercise professionals. If they have specialized PD training or education, hopefully, but not necessarily, they will list that on their profile at the registry. This registry includes professionals with ASC, ASCM, National Council on Strength and Fitness (NCSF), National Strength and Conditioning Association (NSCA), and National Council for Certified Personal Trainers (NCCPT) credentials. Go to usreps.org.

Parkinson's Foundation Establishes Gold-Standard Evaluation and Accreditation for PD-Specific Exercise Professionals, Programs, and Continuing Education Courses

Most of the time, your doctor will send you to local PD websites listing various programs. However, just because a program is listed does not mean the people shown on the site as trainers are qualified, so you mustn't just assume those programs have people with the right credentials to work with you.

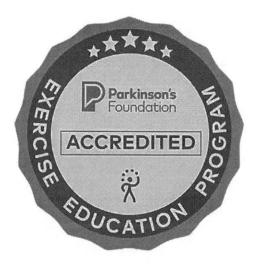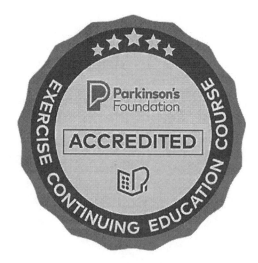

Figure 6: When you see the Parkinson's Foundation (PF) Exercise Education program seal, or the Exercise Continuing Education Course seal, you'll know that the program or course has passed a rigorous evaluation to become Parkinson's Foundation accredited.

Exercise coaching and teaching PWPD requires specialized training that is usually offered through diverse programs to educate exercise professionals who work with PWPD. However, until recent years, there has been no gold standard to define criteria for PD exercise training programs to ensure that their participants (exercise professionals) become competent in working with PWPD. This has led to variability in skills among exercise professionals, as well as uncertainty for PWPD and healthcare providers when they evaluate the safety and effectiveness of PD exercise programs.

Use Exercise Programs and Courses Accredited through the Parkinson's Foundation

The Parkinson's Foundation Exercise Accreditation Recognition distinguishes PD-specific exercise education programs and courses that align with and adhere to the Foundation's Criteria for Exercise Education (see Appendix B) and its Competency Framework for Exercise Professionals (see Appendix C).

Chapter 11

Parkinson's Foundation Exercise Education Programs

These programs have met the rigorous requirements of the Parkinson's Foundation Exercise Competency Framework. These comprehensive programs provide and assess knowledge and skill acquisition, allowing participants to become accredited exercise professionals in the specific program. Participants are assessed on an ongoing basis to maintain certification.

Among the most notable PD specialty program certifications are:

Movement Revolution
Certification offers a Neuro Exercise Specialist training program
movement-revolution.com

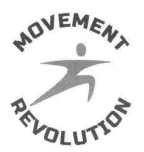

PWR!Moves Certification
pwr4life.org

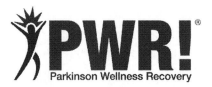

Rock Steady Boxing Certification.
Go to rocksteadyboxing.org

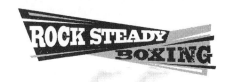

Parkinson's Foundation Continuing Education Courses

The organizations that provide these courses have met the requirement of aligning their curriculum with the Foundation's competency standards. Each course provides knowledge and skills of a particular competency standard. These courses fulfill a continuing education requirement for a certified exercise professional—attendees do not receive a certification or title upon completion, but rather a certificate.

Among the most notable continuing education courses:

MDT Education Solutions
movementdisorderstraining.com

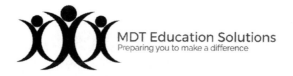

Total HealthWorks continuing education courses
totalhealthworks.com

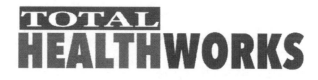

Free Educational Parkinson's Course

American Parkinson Disease Association (APDA)
Parkinson's Training Certificate course for fitness professionals
apdaparkinson.org/pd-fitness-training

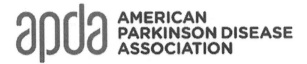

NCCA Approved Parkinson's Programs and Courses

ACE-Approved Parkinson's Cycling Coach
for currently certified training professionals
Go to parkinsonscyclingcoach.com

ACE-ACSM-Approved Urban Poling
Go to urbanpoling.com

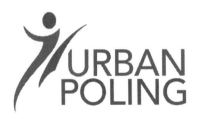

Additional Resources

If you need further assistance with finding someone in your area who works with PWPD or want more information on PD, contact any of the following PD organizations.

The American Parkinson's Disease Association

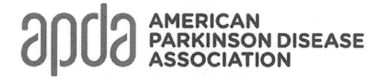

Founded in 1961, APDA has raised and invested more than $252 million to provide outstanding patient services and educational programs, elevate public awareness about the disease, and support research designed to unlock the mysteries of PD and ultimately put an end to this disease. To learn more about the support, programs, and resources APDA provides nationally through its network of Chapters and Information & Referral Centers, as well as its Research Program and Centers for Advanced Research, get in touch with the APDA Team.

800-223-2732
apdaparkinson.org

The Davis Phinney Foundation for Parkinson's

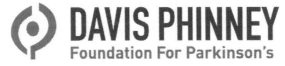

The Davis Phinney Foundation was created in 2004, by Olympic medalist and retired professional cyclist Davis Phinney to help people with PD live well today. The
Foundation's focus is to provide programs and resources that offer inspiration,
information, and tools that help people living with PD take action that can immediately improve their quality of life. Two of the most comprehensive books on Parkinson's disease—the Every Victory Counts Manual and the Every Victory Counts
Manual for Care Partners—are available through their website.

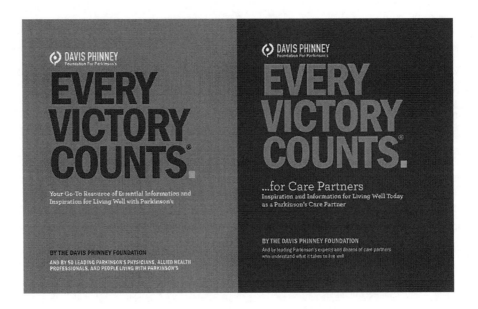

**The Every Victory Counts Manual and the Every Victory Counts Manual for Care
Partners are available through their website at www.dpf.org.**

1-866-358-0285
dpf.org

The Michael J. Fox Foundation for Parkinson's Research

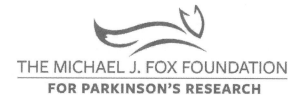

As the world's largest nonprofit funder of PD research, The Michael J. Fox Foundation (MJFF) is dedicated to accelerating a cure for PD and improved therapies for those living with the condition today. The Foundation pursues its goals through an aggressively funded, highly targeted research program coupled with active global engagement of scientists, PD patients, business leaders, clinical trial participants, donors and volunteers. In funding more than $1.75 billion in research programs to date, MJFF has fundamentally altered the trajectory of progress toward a cure.

Instagram: @michaeljfoxorg
Facebook: @michaeljfoxfoundation
Twitter/X: @michaeljfoxorg
LinkedIn: @The Michael J. Fox Foundation for Parkinson's Research
michaeljfox.org

Chapter 11

Parkinson's Foundation

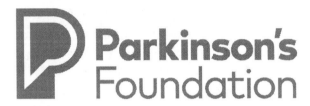

The Parkinson's Foundation makes life better for people with PD by improving care and advancing research toward a cure. In everything they do, they build on the energy, experience, and passion of their global PD community. Since 1957, the Parkinson's Foundation has invested more than $425 million in PD research and clinical care. Their helpline has specialists who can answer your PD questions and offer local PD expert referrals and resources:

M-F 9:00 a.m. – 7:00 p.m. ET (English and Spanish)
1-800-4PD-INFO (1-800-473-4636)
Helpline@Parkinson.org
Parkinson.org

CHAPTER 12

The Future of PD Exercise

"If you put your mind to it, you can accomplish anything."

– In the words of Marty McFly
(performance by Michael J. Fox, *Back to the Future***)**

PWPD Need Specific Exercise Guidance to Motivate Them

The future of PD exercise depends on motivating PWPD to exercise. What will it take in the future to help get us over this hurdle? In a 2018 review article titled "Mobilizing Parkinson's Disease: The Future of Exercise," the authors review the state of the art in key areas and speculate on the likely state of research in each area in the next twenty years. "Key areas relate to: (1) the physiological benefits of exercise with respect to disease modification; (2) the best type of exercise; (3) the optimal intensity of exercise; and (4) implementation strategies to increase exercise uptake" (Ellis and Rochester S95). Are you ready to pick out the name of your PD Exercise Cocktail Plan™?

The review states that exercise, "It is essential, but not sufficient, for neurologists/physicians to recommend exercise/physical activity as part of the standard treatment for PD. However, simply suggesting to patients that they should exercise does not provide the necessary guidance for most to be successful" (Ellis and Rochester S99). And we all know this is not enough. People need specific and continual changes to their exercise plans as their symptoms change. They also need a coach who provides encouragement and daily feedback, and support from the other PWPD in the group classes that encourage them to come back even on days when they may not feel they want to because PD is making it hard to get there. In the future, that coach may be a physical coach or a virtual real-time coach.

> **People [PWPD] need specific and continual changes to their exercise plans as their symptoms change. They also need a coach who provides encouragement and daily feedback, and support from the other PWPD in the group classes that encourage them to come back even on days when they may not feel they want to because PD is making it hard to get there.**
>
> **- Dr. Terry Ellis**

Chapter 12

Smartphone and Tablet Technologies with Feedback and Goal Setting Are in the Works

At this time, PD physical therapists and exercise professionals who work with PWPD (and who also work in concert with the neurologists) are uniquely positioned to help create PD Exercise Cocktail Plans™ with the type and amount of exercise required to effect change for PWPD.

First, however, these professionals should understand the exercise guidelines that have been scientifically proven to help effect symptom change, as discussed in this book. PD Exercise Cocktail Plans™ will then have an immediate impact on PWPD's lives. These plans enable professionals to make positive changes now, while we wait for the individualized prescription plans that scientists are working to develop.

Mobile Health Technologies May Be the Future for PD Treatment

Technology offers a solution to many PWPD, who, for various reasons, have limited access to physical therapists, exercise coaches, and even neurologists. The one good outcome of the COVID-19 pandemic was the breakdown of previous technology barriers—particularly telemedicine. What we have today are "Internet-connected mHealth [mobile health] tools [that] include mobile telecommunications between medical professionals and their patients. Smartphones, for example, enable text messaging, conference calls with video, instructional video recordings, and visual and spoken feedback between patients and investigators, therapists, or a social support group. In addition, wearable sensors with algorithms that recognize activity patterns can identify the type, quantity, and aspects of quality of movements during skills practice and daily activities" (Dobkin "Rehabilitation" 220).

According to researchers Ellis and Rochester, "Advances in mobile health (mHealth) technologies offer a potential solution to help people with PD engage in physical activity and exercise successfully while staying connected to a physiotherapist or healthcare professional. For example, a set of home-based Rehabilitation Internet-of-Things (RIoT) has the potential to optimize exercise uptake and increase physical activity. A RIoT could include wearable, activity recognition sensors and instrumented rehabilitation devices (i.e., virtual reality systems) that transmit information to a smartphone or tablet regarding the quantity and quality of exercise. Using telerehabilitation approaches, data could be monitored by a healthcare professional and interpreted regularly allowing tailored and timely adaptations to an exercise program. Exercises could be uploaded through smartphone applications ('apps') to provide the necessary 'just right' challenge for each patient based on the data received. Strategies to facilitate behavioral change (i.e., goal setting, feedback, rewards) could be provided through apps to foster a more active lifestyle. PWPD could also be connected to others from around the world to provide support, comradery, or friendly competitions to increase engagement, both socially and physically. These types of approaches will likely be more mainstream in the future with the goal of improving exercise/physical activity uptake" (Ellis and Rochester S99).

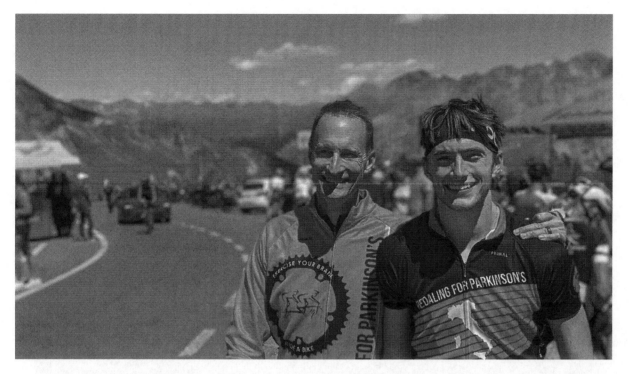

Dr. Jay Alberts, left, takes his research to heart and is an avid cyclist. In 2022, he and his son, Grant, rode the famed Stelvio Pass through the Italian Alps with a group of cyclists from the Davis Phinney Foundation for Parkinson's. During the week of this photo, they rode between 40 and 60 miles a day at 6000 ft. Wearing Dr. Albert's non-profit organization Pedaling for Parkinson's apparel, they rode daily in their PFP gear.

The most significant factor for success regarding symptom management and disease progression is each person with PD. All the beautiful news in this book doesn't help anyone if you don't get up and move. We have given research, inspirational stories, and knowledge to arm you on your PD exercise journey. "Does exercise have significant promise to mitigate the burden and possibly the course of PD? We think so. But to answer that question we will need to design trials that account for the multisystem nature of PD, identify the specific effects of exercise and target the underlying pathophysiology/mechanisms. A better understanding of this would allow for a more personalized approach rather than the current 'one size fits all' and could most likely confer greater benefits. It's no good of course if you don't do it! So embedding exercise in an individual's lifestyle, while accounting for their preferences and ability will most likely enhance uptake and compliance. As we move further into the digital age, supporting technologies will supplement and facilitate delivery from the earliest stage (prodromal) through to later stages of PD adapting to individuals needs on the way. We hope that future research will target these aspects and bring exercise and an active lifestyle as one of the primary tools for clinical management and patient benefit" (Ellis and Rochester S99).

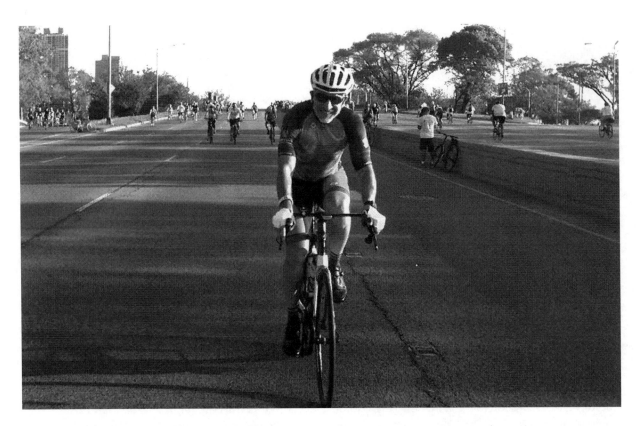

Professor Daniel Corcos, cycling on Lake Shore Drive in Chicago. To keep up with his demanding schedule. He bikes and strength-trains daily. His patients know that he religiously "walks the talk."

The PD Exercise Future Is, as the Timbuk3 Song Says, "So Bright I Gotta Wear Shades"

When I interviewed our three distinguished scientists—Dr. Alberts, Professor Corcos, and Professor Bloem—I asked them each to share what the future of PD exercise looked like. Dr. Alberts said that in the future, he would have a predictive model that tells PWPD what they will achieve by exercising. For example, a person with PD would give their demographics, disease history, medications, etc. Then, someone would enter this data into a modeling computer system. Combinations of the data and nomograms (mathematical devices that show relationships between variables) would predict how much decrease in motor symptoms the PWPD would have after a given amount of time (e.g., twelve months) of performing high-intensity exercise. Knowing precisely the expected symptom results they would achieve ahead of time would empower PWPD and give them hope. It would also increase their motivation and belief in their ability to exercise.

Professor Corcos Predicts Treadmills for PWPD and Custom Blood Profiles That Tell Each Person Exactly How to Counter PD Symptoms through Exercise

Professor Corcos predicted after SPARX3 that he could envision an insurance company providing a treadmill for everybody with PD who wanted one—particularly with the large numbers of newly diagnosed PWPD

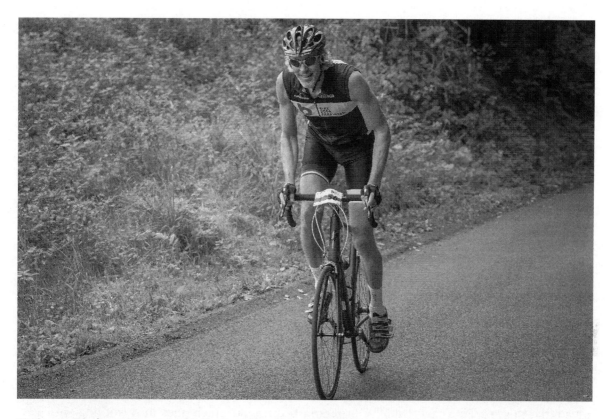

Professor Bastiaan Bloem, cycling in the hills of The Netherlands, puts into practice what he tells his patients to do—exercise at 80% of maximum heart rate at least three days a week. However, he tells them to plan on exercising daily. His rationale is that if they plan on only working out three days a week, they will only get in one workout when life gets in the way. So, it's better to plan on working out daily and get in three days.

expected by 2030. If these new PWPD followed the SPARX3 protocol from day one, it would significantly impact their lives for the better. Professor Corcos also foresaw the potential of having blood-derived biomarker data that could go with Dr. Albert's exercise prescription. Professor Corcos said, "I hope that in a few years when PWPD get their exercise prescription, they would also get their blood profile, and it would say, perhaps, that the reactive protein is high—an index of inflammation. And we know we need to get that down, and exercise brings it down, so I think we're getting there."

Professor Bloem Says It's Time That Doctors Wrote Prescriptions for Exercise

There is undoubtedly enough science behind PD exercise for doctors and insurance companies to recognize that it works to help PWPD manage their symptoms. I asked Professor Bloem what he saw for the future of PD exercise. He responded, "How much more evidence do we need before a doctor, instead of prescribing levodopa, writes an exercise prescription? And I think we've come to that stage, and it's not either, but you need both. So, I'm not against drugs per se, but I'm a great fan of exercise for all the reasons mentioned throughout this book—you need both."

Chapter 12

"Another piece of advice that I would like to give to PWPD," said Professor Bloem, "Is don't be afraid of the medication either. And if you are severely debilitated by Parkinson's, medication can bring you up to the next level where you can then begin to exercise. So, it's the interaction between the medication and the exercise that gives you the greatest benefit. The time has come for doctors like myself to no longer just prescribe medication; we need to prescribe exercise as well and, indeed, lifestyle interventions in general."

The Future Holds a Parkinson's Exercise Specialist Certification Accredited by an NCCA National Organization

My prediction for the future of PD exercise is the establishment of an NCCA-accredited agency Parkinson's Exercise Specialist Certification. An NCCA agency will work with the Parkinson's Foundation to create a certification to meet all the criteria defined by the Competency Framework recently developed by the Parkinson's Foundation. It will be a process similar to when the American College of Exercise built its Cancer Exercise Specialist certification with the American Cancer Society. When that happens, PWPD can look in the U.S. Registry of Exercise Professionals (usreps.org) for the names of people who hold certifications and see their credentials and years of experience, as well as where and how to find these accredited professionals.

It's Our Job as Exercise Professionals to Create Experiences

I would also like to see a PD coach training program, because so much goes into working with PWPD that is not just about teaching a class but rather about creating an experience. The experience should be so encompassing that PWPD cannot wait to return and participate in the next adventure. Every "event," whether it's boxing, cycling, dance, or yoga, should be filled with joy, wonder, fun, effort, and support from the people around them—then the exercise doesn't feel like exercise.

As exercise professionals who work with PWPD, it's our job to give our people that experience every time they step into the room. Remember that this may be, for some, the highlight of their week and the only thing they have to look forward to.

Exercise Is Your New Job—Do What You Love

My message to people with neurological diseases is that "exercise is your new job." For the benefit of care partners and those living around PWPD, the best thing that anyone living with PD can do is work to help manage, stabilize, and hopefully reduce their own symptoms. That requires commitment. Find a program or class nearby and go watch. See what it's all about. Take it all in and try everything.

As I mentioned, many people I've worked with didn't think they would like boxing and now they love it—the same goes for cycling, tai chi, dancing and so on. Start gradually, work up to recommended levels and intensities, and rely on a group of fellow PWPD to motivate and support you.

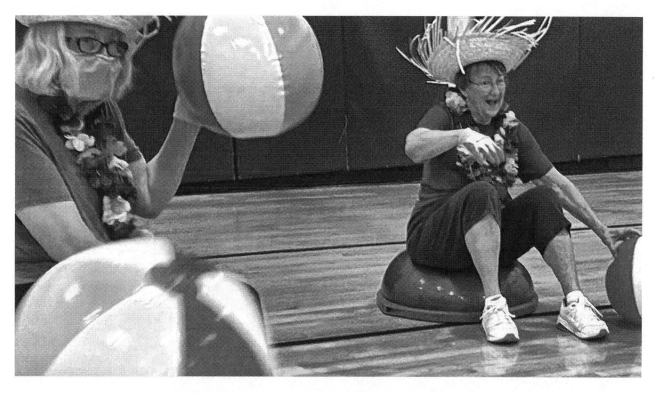

During a Total HealthWorks' Total Parkinson's Class, it's an "Aloha Beach" theme day. Sandy Trent, left, and Linda O'Hair are sitting on BOSU® balls using their abdominal muscles for stability while they call out the names of flowers when they throw the ball to another participant. Creating experiences in the classroom is crucial for exercise professionals. Taking the time to add surprise events makes exercise fun, and PWPD are eager to return and participate in the next adventure.

"Let's Just Exercise!"

Remember my client Linda O'Hair, who was a care partner to her husband with PD for twenty years and then was diagnosed with PD herself? Despite that, she is the one who rallies the troops. She says, "I'm not going to let Parkinson's beat me, and exercise is the only way I can do it. There aren't any medications yet that are going to cure it, so let's just exercise!"

APPENDIX A

The Parkinson's Foundation strives to add more PD Programs and CEC Courses that apply for the selection process in whichever category they choose. If an organization passes the accreditation process, they join others already listed on the Parkinson's Foundation website. So, keep an eye on their website as the number of accredited programs and approved courses grows. Read about the Parkinson's s Foundation criteria for programs below.

Criteria for Exercise Education Programs

These expectations collectively outline how programs educate and train exercise professionals to apply their existing knowledge and skills.

The organization of these expectations into five domains is intended to aid interpretation. Each describes important components that, in combination with their existing expertise, help education programs and CE Courses develop their curriculum to teach the competencies for exercise professionals.

1 Parkinson's Disease: Foundational Information on the Diagnosis, Treatment, and the Role of Exercise

Criteria for Exercise Education Programs

a. Programs are designed to provide basic education on Parkinson's including topics such as the following: what defines Parkinson's (differential diagnoses, related neurological diseases, comorbidities), how it is diagnosed, demographics of the Parkinson's population (e.g., age, gender, race), stages of the disease, disease progression, and symptoms (including motor and non-motor).

b. Programs are designed to provide basic education on the treatment for people with Parkinson's disease which includes medical management, surgical interventions, rehabilitation therapies, psychosocial support, and exercise.

c. Programs are designed to provide basic education on the roles and scopes of practice of the interprofessional care team.

d. Programs are designed to provide education on the evidence-based benefits of exercise for people with Parkinson's (health, neurological, physical, social, emotional) and potential barriers (risk of injury, other complications).

e. Programs are designed to provide education about developing engaging interpersonal relationships with people with Parkinson's and their care partners including the psychosocial dynamics of these interactions.

2 Screening for People with Parkinson's Disease to Participate in Exercise

Criteria for Exercise Education Programs

a. Programs are designed to provide education on Parkinson's-specific health-risk screening and documentation (e.g., health history, fitness goals, medical release, current/past activity, exercise restrictions/contraindications, liability waiver/release) for different exercise options prior to exercise participation.

b. Programs are designed to provide instruction on conducting physical assessments (e.g., aerobic fitness, muscular strength and endurance, movement assessment, including balance, agility, flexibility, and posture assessments) required for the exercise plan prior to participation.

Reprinted with permission from the Parkinson's Foundation 2023

c. Programs are designed to provide guidance on identifying exercise options for people with Parkinson's considering their abilities (e.g., motor, non-motor), safety and health risks, practical feasibility (e.g., location, economics, stage of the disease), and personal goals.

3 Group/Individual Exercise Design for People with Parkinson's Disease

Criteria for Exercise Education Programs

a. Programs are designed to provide training on development of exercise plans for people with Parkinson's that include modifications, adaptations, progressions, and regressions.

b. Programs are designed to cover each domain of exercise specified by the Parkinson's Foundation Exercise Guidelines, if not directly through their program, then by understanding what additional domains could be recommended to people with Parkinson's.

c. Programs are designed to teach participants about creating and maintaining a safe environment for exercise (e.g., facility/home/outdoor fall or trip hazards) by considering Parkinson's-specific safety risks and how to respond to medical and safety incidence that occur during class.

d. Programs are designed to teach participants how to cue, teach, and model exercises to facilitate safe and effective movement for people with Parkinson's.

e. Programs are designed to teach participants how to break down movement sequences through modifications (i.e., progression and regression) in accordance with the Parkinson's Foundation Exercise Guidelines.

4 Exercise Leadership for People with Parkinson's Disease: Human Behavior and Counseling

Criteria for Exercise Education Programs

a. Programs are designed to prepare participants to continuously monitor diverse ability levels to optimize performance and safety which may include modeling, verbal and visual cueing, and modifications (e.g., progression and regression) in accordance with the Parkinson's Foundation Exercise Guidelines.

b. Programs are designed to teach participants how to encourage people with Parkinson's to exercise with optimal movement and at appropriate intensity (physical and cognitive), considering any deconditioning, injuries, or comorbidities.

c. Programs are designed to teach participants how to monitor for safety issues based on Parkinson's-specific risk factors (e.g., functional mobility deficits, freezing of gait, orthostatic hypotension, "Off" time, dyskinesias, Deep Brain Stimulation [DBS], cognitive impairment, mental health) that can lead to falls or other adverse events.

d. Programs are designed to teach participants behavior change strategies (e.g., goal setting, motivation, sense of membership, sense of community, social support) to facilitate engagement and program adherence.

e. Programs are designed to teach participants that they will experience challenges (e.g., disease progression and loss, teaching to a wide variety of ability levels) and rewards (e.g., building self-efficacy/self-confidence, developing resilience, self-advocacy, improved quality of life and mobility) when working with people with Parkinson's.

f. Programs are designed to teach participants about factors impacting their legal risk as an exercise professional and ways to minimize their risk (e.g., liability insurance, waivers, staying within scope of practice, record keeping, confidentiality).

g. Programs are designed to teach participants to refer people with Parkinson's to members of the interprofessional care team and evidence-based resources to answer questions that are outside the participant's scope of practice (e.g., medical questions or treatments, surgical management, onset of pain, falling, freezing of gait, nutrition, sleep, constipation).

5 Interprofessional Communication and Program Development

Criteria for Exercise Education Programs

a. Programs will encourage participants to build relationships and collaborate with other health and wellness providers in the community.

b. Programs will support participants in understanding how to leverage existing community resources to help establish or support Parkinson's-specific community-based classes.

c. Programs will design and implement continuous improvement processes.

These competencies have been released as a pre-print and are currently undergoing scientific peer review. Updates will be posted as the competencies and supporting manuscript are refined for publication.

April 2023

APPENDIX B

Find the Right Path to Further Your Knowledge and Expertise as a Professional Working with PWPD

Before investing your time and money into any PD Program or Continuing Education Unit (CEU) course, ensure that it's the right one. Not all certifications or continuing education courses align with the Parkinson's Foundation's Competency Framework for Exercise Professionals.

Since 2022, the Parkinson's Foundation has exercise education programs and courses accredited by adherence to the competency standards set by the Parkinson's Foundation. "Programs have met the rigorous requirements of the Parkinson's Foundation Exercise Competency Framework. These comprehensive programs provide and assess knowledge and skill acquisition, allowing participants to become accredited exercise professionals."

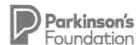

Competency Framework for Exercise Professionals

These expectations collectively outline how exercise professionals design and deliver exercise leadership to people with Parkinson's.

These expectations are divided into five domains intended to aid interpretation. Each describes important components that, in combination with their existing expertise, help exercise professionals achieve competence when working with people with Parkinson's.

1 Parkinson's Disease: Foundational Information on the Diagnosis, Treatment, and the Role of Exercise

1. Apply their basic understanding of Parkinson's to discuss the range of symptoms and treatments with a person with Parkinson's and their care partners.
2. Understand the impact of a Parkinson's diagnosis and treatment on quality of life, and the potential for exercise to enhance a range of health and quality of life outcomes for people with Parkinson's.
3. Awareness of basic effects and complications of common treatments used for Parkinson's and co-morbid conditions that impact a person with Parkinson's disease such as their physiological response to, or ability to participate in exercise.
4. Understand how Parkinson's disease, as well as other co-morbidities, can increase an individual's risk of injury and other complications from exercise.

2 Screening for People with Parkinson's Disease to Participate in Exercise

1. Select health-risk screening and physical assessments as appropriate for the exercise plan.
2. Evaluate the screening results to determine if a person with Parkinson's is presumed reasonably safe to participate in the exercise program prior to conducting any physical assessments (relevant to the program).
3. Identify and/or create appropriate exercise options/plans for people with Parkinson's considering their abilities (e.g., motor, non-motor), safety and health risks, practical feasibility (e.g., location, economics, stage of the disease), and personal goals.

3 Group/Individual Exercise Design for People with Parkinson's Disease

1. Design exercise plans by:
    a. selecting and ordering exercises with disease-specific considerations (e.g., extended warm-up, range of motion, attention to heart rate, recovery time).
    b. incorporating the domains of fitness in accordance with the Parkinson's Exercise Guidelines.
    c. considering other Parkinson's-related factors (e.g., cognitive/emotional, functional skills, ADLs) and challenges (e.g., stooped posture, balance/weight-shifting, axial rotation, transitions/multi-directional stepping, gait, rigidity, non-motor symptoms).

Reprinted with permission from the Parkinson's Foundation 2023

2. Select appropriate equipment based on the exercise plan and implement safety protocols as needed given Parkinson's-specific safety risks.
3. Understand how to modify class design considering instructor/exercise client ratios and accommodations for disease progression (e.g., participation of care partners) including the accommodation of several ability levels within the same class.
4. Respond to medical and safety incidents occurring during class, including distinguishing between emergency and non-emergency situations.

4 Exercise Leadership for People with Parkinson's Disease: Human Behavior and Counseling

1. Demonstrate exercise activities for people with Parkinson's including teaching, cueing and modeling exercises, modifying exercises through progressions and regressions while monitoring and adjusting for potential safety risks.
2. Adapt exercise instruction as necessary for individual or class sessions (e.g., speak louder, demonstrate several modifications of the same exercise, use expanded cueing and modeling techniques).
3. Identify teachable moments for people with Parkinson's and take that opportunity to provide appropriate information and education.
4. Apply strategies that promote behavior change (e.g., goal setting, motivation, sense of membership, sense of community, social support) to facilitate engagement and program adherence.
5. Recognize when changes in the health status (motor or non-motor symptoms, injuries, surgeries) of a person with Parkinson's warrant a referral to another member of the interprofessional care team or to a more appropriate exercise or movement option.
6. Mitigate legal risk and apply their understanding of responsibilities as an exercise professional (e.g., liability insurance, waivers, staying within scope of practice, incident reporting, when medical clearance is required or needs to be revisited).

5 Interprofessional Communication and Program Development

1. Understand how to build and maintain an interprofessional care network of individuals who work with people with Parkinson's and understand the scope of practice of each type of professional.
2. Encourage people with Parkinson's to visit their physical therapist on a regular basis for initial and re-evaluation.
3. Encourage people with Parkinson's to seek appropriate care from physicians and other members of the interprofessional care team as appropriate given their Parkinson's-specific motor and non-motor symptoms, and general health concerns.
4. Understand how to incorporate care partners and other assistants into the exercise plan to increase success and safety.

These competencies have been released as a pre-print and are currently undergoing scientific peer review. Updates will be posted as the competencies and supporting manuscript are refined for publication.

April 2023

APPENDIX C

Selected National Commission for Certifying Agencies (NCCA) Accredited Certification Agencies 2023

The following top-tier fitness agencies are in addition to the ones mentioned in Chapter 11. These organizations have been accredited by the NCCA and issue Certified Personal Trainer and/or Group Exercise Fitness certifications.

American College of Sports Medicine (ACSM), acsm.org

- NCCA Personal Trainer

National Exercise and Sports Trainers Association (NESTA), nestacertified.com

- NCCA Personal Trainer

National Exercise Trainers Association (NETA), netafit.org

- NCCA Personal Trainer Certification
- NCCA Group Exercise

National Federation of Professional Trainers (NFPT), www.nfpt.com

- NCCA Personal Trainer Certification

National Strength and Conditioning Association (NSCA), www.nsca.com

- NCCA Personal Trainer certification

National Council on Strength and Fitness (NCSF), www.ncsf.org

- NCCA Personal Trainer certification

ACRONYM LIST

ACE	American Council on Exercise
ACSM	American College of Sports Medicine
ADL	activities of daily living
ACSM	American College of Sports Medicine
APDA	American Parkinson's Disease Association
BBB	blood-brain barrier
BOLD	blood oxygen level dependent
BDNF	brain-derived neurotrophic factor
CEC	continuing education course
CNS	central nervous system
CPT	Certified Personal Trainer
COVID-19	coronavirus pandemic 2019
DPF	Davis Phinney Foundation for Parkinson's
FE	forced-effort (pedaling at a rate faster than you normally would)
GFI	Group Fitness Instructor
MHR	maximum heart rate
NASM	National Academy of Sports Medicine
NCCA	The National Commission for Certifying Agencies
NSCA	The National Strength and Conditioning Association
PD	Parkinson's Disease
PFP	Pedaling for Parkinson's™

ACRONYM LIST

PFP	Pedaling for Parkinson's™
PRE	perceived rate of exertion
PRE	progressive resistance exercise
PSP	Progressive Supranuclear Palsy
PT	physical therapist
PWPD	person or people with Parkinson's disease
RAGBRAI	Register's Annual Great Bicycle Ride Across Iowa
RIoT	Rehabilitation Internet-of-Things
RPE	rate of perceived exertion
RPM	revolutions per minute
RSB	Rock Steady Boxing
SPARX2	Study in Parkinson's Disease of Exercise Phase 2 (Treadmill)
SPARX3	Study in Parkinson's Disease of Exercise Phase 3 (Treadmill)
THW	Total HealthWorks
VE	voluntary effort (pedaling at their own pace)

ACKNOWLEDGEMENTS

I give special thanks to Jay Alberts, with whom I have had the privilege of working for seven years. We have often talked about the need for this book, but in 2021 when I mentioned actually sitting down and writing it, I'm not sure he believed I would do it. However, several months later, when I started sending him drafts, he was surprised and thrilled that it would finally become a reality.

I appreciate Daniel Corcos, who was gracious with his time, knowledge, and belief in this book. He is a wellspring of knowledge and expertise, and we had a wonderful time debating crucial concepts during the many iterations of the manuscript.

Many thanks to Bas Bloem for his invaluable insights and writing the foreword of the book. He was so excited that the book was being written, and I will never forget him saying, "This book is long overdue."

Without my incredible development editor, Dan Janal, I could not have written this book. Dan made my work shine much brighter and clearer, and he truly loved its purpose and intent—I can't thank Dan enough.

Cliff Lawson truly saved the day for me. We have worked together for over twenty years, and he has been my "editor extraordinaire" on many of my published works. Once again, Cliff went through my manuscript and worked his magic to make my book more focused and concise without losing my writing style—he is the best at what he does. I'm so incredibly grateful to Cliff and happy to have had such an amazing person in my life.

Larry Butler was a joy to work with; he is a meticulous copyeditor who does exceptional work. So happy to have Larry on my team.

I cannot thank Lucy Spencer enough for her diligence in the final proofing of the book. She was indispensable to its completion. We worked in the early morning hours to get it to print.

I want to thank Dr. Steven Aldeman, DO, Neurology, with whom I have worked for years, for providing feedback in the early stages of this book that led to the development of Chapter 11. That chapter contains essential information on finding a qualified exercise professional who works with PWPD.

Lisa Hoffman at the Parkinson's Foundation was a fountain of expertise and knowledge. I greatly appreciated working with her to define the previously uncharted landscape of exercise professionals who work with PWPD. Thank you, Lisa.

ACKNOWLEDGEMENTS

Thanks to Bill Roach, my mentor and dear friend, who taught me about PD and how to work with PWPD. I certainly wouldn't be where I am today if it were not for Bill.

I can never thank Jane Collison enough for her unending support not only to me but to my Parkinson's work. She is always behind the scenes working her magic. She truly makes the Parkinson's community a better place with all that she contributes to the people in it.

Kay Arvidson was such a support to me during the writing of this book that I cannot thank her adequately for the wisdom and insight she so graciously shared with me throughout this process.

Many thanks to Linda O'Hair who patiently listened to me wrestle with the difficulties of writing this book. Linda would listen and smile and assure me it would all work out. And I believed her. Thank you, Linda.

I would like to thank our partners at the Grand Living at Tower Place, an assisted-living facility in West Des Moines, Iowa, for their support of my book, my Parkinson's work, and of the Parkinson's community.

A special thanks to the Davis Phinney Foundation's Ambassador Leadership Program Team. They put together an amazing annual September 2022 Leadership Conference that inspired me to immediately start writing this book. One year later, the final draft manuscript was complete.

I thank my clients who have shared their lives with me through many years and who are now helping others by sharing their PD stories: Joe and Gail Johll, Jane Collison and Bob McCracken, Carol Harvey, Sandy Trent, Bill Brown, Kay Arvidson, Joe Hingl, Julie Aufdenkamp, Linda O'Hair, Jim Best, Kim Beisser, Mike Hawkins, and Joyce Gamble.

Thanks to all the wonderful PWPD that I interviewed for the book, who shared their incredible PD journeys. I thank Cidney and Pat Donahoo, John Tomeny, Rhonda Foulds, John Ball, DawnElla Rust, Trent MacLean, John Cullen, Tom and Chris Timberlake, Joe Mende, and Steve Gilbert.

Many thanks to the readers of my first draft who took the time to read and share insights: Professor Daniel Corcos, PhD; Professor Baastian Bloem, PhD, MD, FRCPE; Dr. Steve Alderman, DO; Dr. Jim Collison, MD; Kathy Helmuth, RN; Dr. Steven Zhang, MD; Linda K. Olsen, MD; Dr. Stephanie A. Miller, PT, PhD, NCS; Dr. Mike Collison, MD; Kristy Rose Follmar, Scott Newman, Jane Collison, Bob McCracken, Carol Harvey, Sandy Trent, Bill Brown, Kay Arvidson, Joe Hingl, Julie Aufdenkamp, Wade Collison, Margaret Collison, Linda O'Hair, Jim Best, Katie Collison, Kim Beisser, Mike Hawkins, Joyce Gamble, Cidney and Pat Donahoo, Richard Collison, John Tomeny, Rhonda Foulds, John Ball, DawnElla Rust, Trent MacLean, John Cullen, Tom Timberlake, Chris Timberlake, Joe Mende, Steve Gilbert, John Watson, Vilma Calix, John Collison, Thomas Cosentino, Cam Hals, Dan Collison, Brianna Coy, Barbara Dirks, Jerry Gamble, Molly Shonsey, Alden Collison, and Bill Roach.

BIOGRAPHIES

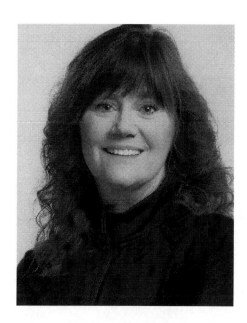

Kristine Meldrum

Photo by Bob Ocken

Kristine Meldrum is the author of *Parkinson's: How to Reduce Symptoms Through Exercise*. She is an exercise professional working with PD patients and other neurological clients. She is the Founder and President of Parkinson's Place, Iowa, and writes and speaks nationally at Parkinson's Conferences with a presentation titled *How to Exercise to Improve Parkinson's Symptoms*. Kristine has spent fifteen years in the fitness industry and worked a decade in the medical-fitness industry before starting a neuro-wellness-program in 2020. Kristine engages one-on-one with clients and teaches neuro classes at The Grand Living at Tower Place in West Des Moines, Iowa. She also consults with organizations to help start neuro wellness programs. Contact her for speaking engagements and book sales

BIOGRAPHIES

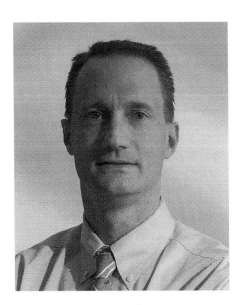

JAY ALBERTS

Jay L. Alberts, PhD, is the Vice Chair of Innovations within the Neurological Institute at the Cleveland Clinic, holder of the Edward F. and Barbara A. Bell Family Endowed Chair, staff member with the Department of Biomedical Engineering and also holds an appointment in the Department of Biomedical Engineering at the Cleveland Clinic. He has worked extensively in the development of exercise for individuals with PD. Dr. Alberts has written 100+ peer-reviewed journal articles and speaks globally on PD, technology, virtual reality, and PD exercise. Dr. Alberts founded Pedaling for Parkinson's, a non-profit organization for PWPD. Contact Jay for speaking engagements through kristinemeldrum@parkinsonsplaceiowa.org.

BIOGRAPHIES

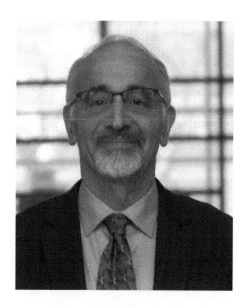

DANIEL M. CORCOS

Daniel M. Corcos, PhD, is a professor in the Department of Physical Therapy & Human Movement Sciences at the Feinberg School of Medicine and a Professor in the McCormick School of Engineering at Northwestern University. He has published extensively on the treatments for PD and how the treatments work. He has published influential papers on strength and endurance training for PWPD. He was responsible for the section on PD in the American College of Sports Medicine's Guidelines for Exercise Testing and Prescription, 11th Edition. Dr. Corcos has written 200+ peer-reviewed journal articles and speaks globally on PD and the exercise prescription for PD exercise. Contact Daniel for speaking engagements through kristinemeldrum@parkinsonsplaceiowa.org.

WORKS CITED

Please Note: MLA 9 adds a period at the end of a URL. It is not part of the original URL, so copy it correctly if you look up a cited work.

Abbott, Robert, et al. "Midlife Milk Consumption and Substantia Nigra Neuron Density at Death." *Neurology*, vol. 86, no. 6, 9 Feb. 2016, pp. 512–9. https://doi:10.1212/WNL.0000000000002254.

American Council on Exercise, "What is Accreditation?" *acefitness.org*, https://www.acefitness.org/fitness-certifications/accreditation. Accessed Oct 13, 2022.

Ahlskog, Eric. "Aerobic Exercise: Evidence for a Direct Brain Effect to Slow Parkinson Disease Progression." *Mayo Clinic Proceedings*, vol. 93, no. 3, Mar. 2018, pp. 360–372. https://doi:10.1016/j.mayocp.2017.12.015.

Alberts, Jay L., et al. "It Is Not About the Bike; It Is About the Pedaling: Forced Exercise and Parkinson's Disease." *Exercise and Sport Sciences Reviews*, vol. 39, no. 4, Oct 2011, pp.177–86. https://doi:10.1097/JES.0b013e31822cc71a.

Alberts, Jay L., and Anson Rosenfeldt. "The Universal Prescription for Parkinson's Disease: Exercise." *Journal of Parkinson's Disease*, vol. 10, no. 1, 2020, pp. S21–S27. https://doi:10.3233/JPD-202100.

American Academy of Neurology, "Death Rate from Parkinson's Rising in U.S. Study Finds," 28 Oct. 2021, *ScienceDaily*, https://www.sciencedaily.com/releases/2021/10/211027211902.htm. Accessed 4 Oct. 2022.

American Academy of Neurology. "Pesticide Found in Milk Decades Ago May Be Associated with Signs of Parkinson's." *Science Daily*, 9 Dec. 2015, https://www.sciencedaily.com/releases/2015/12/151209183729.htm. Accessed 5 Oct. 2022.

Anirudhan Athira, et al. "Eleven Crucial Pesticides Appear to Regulate Key Genes That Link MPTP Mechanism to Cause Parkinson's Disease through the Selective Degeneration of Dopamine Neurons." *Brain Science*, vol. 13, no.7, 28 June 2023, pp. 1–16. https://doi:10.3390/brainsci13071003.

Back to the Future. Directed by Robert Zemeckis, performance by Michael J. Fox, Universal Studios, 1985.

Balci, Birgül, et al. "Impact of the COVID-19 Pandemic on Physical Activity, Anxiety, and Depression in Patients with Parkinson's Disease." *International Journal of Rehabilitation Research*, vol 44, no.2, June 2021, pp. 173–176. https://doi:10.1097/MRR.0000000000000460.

Beall, Erik B., et al. "The Effect of Forced-Exercise Therapy for Parkinson's Disease on Motor Cortex Functional Connectivity." *Brain Connectivity*, vol. 3, no. 2, Apr. 2013, pp. 190–8. https://doi:10.1089/brain.2012.0104.

Blue Cross Blue Shield Association. "Prevalence of Parkinson's Disease Rising in Younger Adults." *Blue Cross Blue Shield*, 22 Oct. 2020, https://www.bcbs.com/the-health-of-america/reports/prevalence-of-parkinsons-disease-rising-younger-adults.

Bloem, Bastiaan R. "Exercise in Parkinson's During COVID-19." *Parkinson's Academy Webinar*, 27 Oct. 2020, https://www.youtube.com/watch?v=FTVNrppK2II. Accessed 8 Nov. 2022.

Bloem, Bastiaan R. "Professor Bastiaan Bloem & Ending Parkinson's." *Davis Phinney Foundation*, 17 Mar 2020, https://davisphinneyfoundation.org/professor-bastiaan-bloem-ending-parkinsons/. Accessed 8 Oct. 2022.

Borrione, Paolo, et al. "Effects of Physical Activity in Parkinson's Disease: A New Tool for Rehabilitation." *World Journal of Methodology*, vol. 4, no. 3, 26 Sep. 2014, pp. 133–43. https://doi:10.5662/wjm.v4.i3.133.

Brown, Terry., et al. "Pesticides and Parkinson's Disease—Is There a Link?" *Environmental Health Perspectives*, vol. 114, no. 2, Feb. 2006, pp. 156–64. https://doi:10.1289/ehp.8095.

Calahorrano-Moreno, Micaela Belen, et al. "Sarcopenia and Dynapenia in Patients with Parkinsonism." *Journal of the American Medical Directors Association*, vol. 17, no. 7, 30 Apr. 2016, pp. 640–6. https://doi:10.12688/f1000research.108779.1.

Calahorrano-Moreno, Micaela Belen, et al. "Contaminants in the Cow's Milk We Consume? Pasteurization and Other Technologies in the Elimination of Contaminants." *F1000 Research*, vol. 11, no. 91, 25 Jan. 2022, pp. 2–34. https://doi:10.12688/f1000research.108779.1.

Caspersen, Carl J., et al. "Physical Activity, Exercise, and Physical Fitness: Definitions and Distinctions for Health-Related Research." *Public Health Reports* (Washington, D.C. 1974), vol.100, no.2, 1985, pp.126–31. https://www.ncbi.nlm.nih.gov/pmc/articles/PMC1424733/.

Charcot, Jean-Martin. "Vibratory Therapeutics. The Application of Rapid and Continuous Vibrtions to the Treatment of Certain Diseases of the Nervous System. 1892." *The Journal of Nervous and Mental Disease*, vol. 199, no.11, 2011, pp. 821–7. https://doi:10.1097/NMD.0b013e31823899bc.

Clark, Brian C., and Todd M. Manini. "What is dynapenia?" *Nutrition*, vol. 28, no. 5, 2012) pp. 1-19. https://doi:10.1016/j.nut.2011.12.002.

Combs, Stephanie A., et al. "Boxing Training for Patients with Parkinson Disease: A Case Series." *Physical Therapy*, vol. 91, no. 1, 1 Jan. 2011, pp. 132–42. https://doi:10.2522/ptj.20100142.

Combs-Miller, Stephanie A. "Fighting Parkinson's." *YouTube*, University of Indianapolis, 27 Feb. 2015, https://www.youtube.com/watch?v=F4Lj6sGMb-I. Accessed 15 Oct. 2022.

Combs-Miller, Stephanie A., and Elizabeth Moore. "Predictors of Outcomes in Exercisers with Parkinson Disease: A Two-Year Longitudinal Cohort Study." *NeuroRehabilitation*, vol. 44, no. 3, 20 June 2019, pp. 425–432. https://doi:10.3233/NRE-182641.

Corcos, Daniel M., et al. "A Two-Year Randomized Controlled Trial of Progressive Resistance Exercise for Parkinson's Disease." *Movement Disorders: Official Journal of the Movement Disorder Society,* vol. 28, no. 9, 27 Mar. 2013, pp.1–19. https://doi:10.1002/mds.

Corcos, Daniel M., et al. "A Two-Year Randomized Controlled Trial of Progressive Resistance Exercise for Parkinson's Disease." Supplementary materials (file name: "NIHMS436737-supplement-Supp_ Material.docx"). In Movement Disorders, vol. 28, no. 9, 27 Mar. 2013. https://doi:10.1002/ mds.

Cohut Maria, "Regular high-intensity exercise may stall Parkinson's symptoms." *Medical News Today*, 17 Dec. 2017, https://www.medicalnewstoday.com/articles/320324. Accessed 15 Oct. 2022.

Destro, Christina. "U.S. Department of Veterans Affairs Expands Benefits for People with Parkinsonism Associated with Agent Orange Exposure." *michaeljfox.org*, 11 Jun 2021, https://www.michaeljfox.org/news/us-department-veterans-affairs-expands-benefits-people-parkinsonism-associated-agent-orange. Accessed 16 Oct. 2022.

Dobkin Bruce H., "A Rehabilitation-Internet-of-Things in the Home to Augment Motor Skills and Exercise Training." *Neurorehabilitation and Neural Repair*, vol. 31, no. 3, 31 Mar. 2017, pp. 217–227. https://doi.org/10.1177/1545968316680490.

Dorsey, E Ray, et al. "The Emerging Evidence of the Parkinson Pandemic." *Journal of Parkinson's Disease*, vol. 8, no. s1, 18 Dec. 2018, pp. S3–S8. https://doi:10.3233/JPD-181474.

Dorsey, Ray, et al. Ending Parkinson's Disease. 1st ed., PublicAffairs, Mar 2020.

Education Department, Parkinson's Foundation, "Fact Sheets: Genetics. Parkinson's Genes." Parkinson's Foundation, https://www.parkinson.org/library/fact-sheets/about-parkinsons. Accessed 6 Oct. 2022.

Ellis, Terry, and Lynn Rochester. "Mobilizing Parkinson's Disease: The Future of Exercise." *Journal of Parkinson's Disease*, vol. 8, no. s1, July 2018, pp. S95–S100. https://doi.org/10.3233/JPD-181489.

Fang, Xuexian, et al. "Association of Levels of Physical Activity with Risk of Parkinson Disease: A Systematic Review and Meta-Analysis." *JAMA Network Open*, vol. 1, no. 5, 21 Sept. 2018, pp.1–11. https://doi:10.1001/jamanetworkopen.2018.2421.

Fisher, Beth E., et al. "The Effect of Exercise Training in Improving Motor Performance and Corticomotor Excitability in People with Early Parkinson's Disease." *Archives of Physical Medicine and Rehabilitation*, vol. 89, no. 7, July 2008, pp. 1221–9. https://doi:10.1016/j.apmr.2008.01.013.

Fragala, Maren S., et al. "Resistance Training for Older Adults: Position Statement from the National Strength and Conditioning Association." *Journal of Strength and Conditioning Research*, vol. 33, no. 8, Aug. 2019, pp. 2019–2052. https://doi:10.1519/JSC.0000000000003230.

Gibson, William R. "Age 65+ Adults Are Projected to Outnumber Children by 2030." *AARP*, 14 Mar. 2018, www.aarp.org/home-family/friends-family/info-2018/census-baby-boomers-fd.html. Accessed 2 Oct. 2022.

Goetz, Christopher G. "Charcot on Parkinson's Disease." *Movement Disorder*, vol. 1, no. 1, 1986, pp. 27–32. https://doi.org/10.1002/mds.870010104. Accessed 6 Oct. 2022.

Gowers, William R., *A Manual of Diseases of the Nervous System*, v.1, 3rd ed., P. Blakiston's Son & Company, 1900, https://www.amazon.com/manual-diseases-nervous-system/dp/B00087UY8S. Accessed 26 Sept. 2022.

Gowers, William R., *A Manual of Diseases of the Nervous System*, v.2, J. & A. Churchill 1886-1888, https://archive.org/details/manualofdiseases02goweuoft.

Greger, Michael. "Why Some Dairy Products Are More Closely Linked to Parkinson's Disease." *Nutrition Facts.org*, 2 July 2019, https://nutritionfacts.org/blog/why-some-dairy-products-are-more-closely-linked-to-parkinsons-disease/. Accessed 01 Oct. 2022.

Herman, Talia, et al. "Six Weeks of Intensve Treadmill Training Improves Gait and Quality of Life in Patients with Parkinson's Disease: A Pilot Study." *Archives of Physical Medicine and Rehabilitation*, vol. 88, no. 9, Sept. 2007, pp. 1154–8. https://doi:10.1016/j.apmr.2007.05.015.

Hicks, Gregory E., et al. "Absolute Strength and Loss of Strength as Predictors of Mobility Decline in Older Adults: the InCHIANTI Study." *The Journals of Gerontology*, vol. 67, no. 1 (2012): pp. 66–73. doi:10.1093/gerona/glr055.

Hughes, Katherine C, et al. "Intake of Dairy Foods and Risk of Parkinson Disease." *Neurology*, vol. 89, no.1, 4 July 2017, pp. 46–52. https://doi:10.1212/WNL.0000000000004057.

Inácio, Patricia. "Pilot Trial of FGF-1 to Promote Blood Vessel Growth in Brain Planned." *Parkinson's News Today*, 17 Jan. 2022, https://parkinsonsnewstoday.com/news/zhittya-plans-pilot-trial-fgf-1-promote-blood-vessel-growth-brain/. Accessed 8 Oct. 2022.

Islam, MD Shahidul, et al. "Pesticides and Parkinson's Disease: Current and Future Perspective." *Journal of Chemical Neuroanatomy*, vol. 115, Sept. 2021, https:// doi:10.1016/j.jchemneu.2021.101966.

Johansson, Hanna, et al. "Exercise-Induced Neuroplasticity in Parkinson's Disease: A Metasynthesis of the Literature." *Neural Plasticity*, vol. 2020, 12 Mar. 2020, pp. 1–15. https://doi:10.1155/2020/8961493.

Johansson, Martin E., et al. "Aerobic Exercise Alters Brain Function and Structure in Parkinson's Disease: A Randomized Controlled Trial." *Annals of Neurology*, vol. 91, no. 2, Feb. 2022, pp. 203–216. https://doi:10.1002/ana.26291.

Kannarkat, George T., et al. "Effect of Exercise and Rehabilitation Therapy on Risk of Hospitalization in Parkinson's Disease." *Movement Disorders Clinical Practice.*" vol. 9, no. 4, 2 May 2022, pp. 494–500. https://doi:10.1002/mdc3.13456.

Kohrt, Wendy M., et al. "Effects of Gender, Age, and Fitness Level on Response of VO2max to Training in 60-71 Yr Old's." *Journal of Applied Physiology*, vol. 71, no. 5, Nov. 1991, pp. 2004–2011. https://10.1152/jappl.1991.71.5.2004

Kumar, David R, et al. "Jean-Martin Charcot: The Father of Neurology." *Clinical Medicine & Research*, vol. 9, no. 1, Mar. 2011, pp. 46–9. https://doi:10.3121/cmr.2009.883.

Larson, Danielle, et al. "High Satisfaction and Improved Quality of Life with Rock Steady Boxing in Parkinson's Disease: Results of a Large-Scale Survey." *Disability and Rehabilitation*, vol. 44, no. 20, Oct. 2022, pp. 6034–6041. https://doi:10.1080/09638288.2021.1963854.

Li, Quanhao, et al. "Tai Chi Versus Routine Exercise in Patients with Early- or Mild-Stage Parkinson's Disease: A Retrospective Cohort Analysis." *Brazilian Journal of Medical and Biological Research = Revista Brasileira de Pesquisas Medicas e Biologicas*, vol. 53, e9171, 10 Feb. 2020, pp. 1–7. https://doi:10.1590/1414-431X20199171.

Liguori, Gary. *ACSM's Guidelines for Exercise Testing and Prescription*. 11th ed., Philadelphia: Lippincott Williams & Wilkins, 2021.

Luxner, Larry. "Dutch Neurologist Warns of 'Parkinson's Pandemic' Linked to Toxic Chemicals." *Parkinson's News Today*, 6 Apr. 2020, https://parkinsonsnewstoday.com/news/dutch-neurologist-bas-bloem-warns-of-parkinsons-pandemic/. Accessed 5 Oct. 2022.

Mahalakshmi, Bharath. et al. "Possible Neuroprotective Mechanisms of Physical Exercise in Neurodegeneration." *International Journal of Molecular Sciences*, vol. 21, no. 16, 2020, pp. 1–17, https://doi:10.3390/ijms21165895.

Mandal, Ananya. "Parkinson's Disease History." *News-Medical-Net*, 04 May 2023, https://www.news-medical.net/health/Parkinsons-Disease-History.aspx. Accessed 5 Oct. 2022.

Miyai, Ichiro, et al. "Long-Term Effect of Body Weight-Supported Treadmill Training in Parkinson's Disease: A Randomized Controlled Trial." *Archives of Physical Medicine and Rehabilitation*, vol. 83, no.10, Oct. 2002, pp. 1370–3. https://doi:10.1053/apmr.2002.34603.

Moore, Abbie, et al. "A Community-based Boxing Program Is Associated with Improved Balance in Individuals with Parkinson's Disease." *International Journal of Exercise Science*, vol. 14, no. 3, 1 June 2021, pp. 876–884. https://www.ncbi.nlm.nih.gov/pmc/articles/PMC8758155/.

Nam, Je Shik, et al. "Hip Fracture in Patients with Parkinson's Disease and Related Mortality: A Population-Based Study in Korea." *Gerontology*, vol. 67, no. 5, 18 Mar. 2021, pp. 544–553. https://doi:10.1159/000513730.

Ozer, Firuzan Fırat, et al. "Sarcopenia, Dynapenia, and Body Composition in Parkinson's Disease: Are They Good Predictors of Disability? A Case-Control Study." *Neurological Sciences: Official Journal of the Italian Neurological Society and of the Italian Society of Clinical Neurophysiology*, vol. 41, no. 2, 3 Oct. 2019, pp. 313–320. https://doi:10.1007/s10072-019-04073-1.

Ovallath, Sujith and Patil Deepa. "The History of Parkinsonism: Descriptions in Ancient Indian Medical Literature." *Movement Disorders*, vol. 28, no. 5, 8 Mar. 2013, pp. 566–568. https://doi.org/10.1002/mds.25420.

Parkinson, James. "An Essay on the Shaking Palsy. 1817." *The Journal of Neuropsychiatry and Clinical Neurosciences*, vol. 14, no. 2, Spring 2002, pp. 223–36; discussion 222. https://doi:10.1176/jnp.14.2.223. Accessed 6 Oct. 2022.

Paul, Marla. "High-intensity exercise delays Parkinson's progression." *Northwestern Now*, 11 Dec. 2011, https://news.northwestern.edu/stories/2017/december/high-intensity-exercise-delays-parkinsons-progression/. Accessed 10 Oct. 2022.

Patterson, Charity, et al. "Study in Parkinson's Disease of Exercise Phase 3 (SPARX3): Study Protocol for a Randomized Controlled Trial." *Trials*, vol. 23, no. 1, 6 Oct. 2022, pp. 1–26. https://doi:10.1186/s13063-022-06703-0.

Pickersgill, Jacob W., et al. "The Combined Influences of Exercise, Diet and Sleep on Neuroplasticity." *Frontiers in Psychology*, vol. 13, Apr. 2022, pp. 1–17. https://doi:10.3389/fpsyg.2022.831819.

Pohl, Marcus, et al. "Immediate Effects of Speed-Dependent Treadmill Training on Gait Parameters in Early Parkinson's Disease." *Archives of Physical Medicine and Rehabilitation*, vol. 84, no. 12, Dec. 2003, pp. 1760–6. https://doi:10.1016/s0003-9993(03)00433-7.

"Posterior Column Ataxia-Retinitis Pigmentosa Syndrome." *Genetic and Rare Diseases Information Center*, Feb 2023, https://rarediseases.info.nih.gov/diseases/9898/posterior-column-ataxia-retinitis-pig mentosa-syndrome. Accessed 10 Oct. 2022.

Radboud University Medical Center. "Exercising at Home Has a Positive Effect on Parkinson's Patients." *Sciencedaily.org*, 12 Sept. 2019. https://www.sciencedaily.com/releases/2019/09/190912112421.htm. Accessed 2 Oct. 2022.

Reed, Paul. "Physical Activity: We All Can and Must Do More." *Health.gov blog*, Office of Disease Prevention and Health Promotion, US Department of Health and Human Services, 16 May 2022, https://health.gov/news/202205/physical-activity-we-all-can-and-must-do-more-0. Accessed 15 Sept. 2022.

"Reviews of Current Literature in Rehabilitation of Persons with Parkinson Disease." *Journal of Neuro-logic Physical Therapy*, vol. 43, no. 1, Jan. 2019, pp. 63–64. https://journals.lww.com/jnpt/Fulltext/2019/01000/Reviews_of_Current_Literature_in_Rehabilitation_of.9.aspx.

Reynolds, Sharon. "Tracking the Spread of Parkinson's Proteins from Gut to Brain." *National Institutes of Health*, U.S. Department of Health and Human Services, 23 July 2019, https://www.nih.gov/news-events/nih-research-matters/tracking-spread-parkinsons-proteins-gut-brain. Accessed 4 Oct. 2022.

Ridgel, Angela, et al. "Dynamic High-Cadence Cycling Improves Motor Symptoms in Parkinson's Disease." *Frontiers in Neurology*, vol. 6, 2015, pp. 1–8. https://doi:10.3389/fneur.2015.00194.

Ridgel, Angela, et al. "Forced, Not Voluntary, Exercise Improves Motor Function in Parkinson's Disease Patients." *Neurorehabilitation and Neural Repair*, vol. 23, no. 6, 8 Jan. 2009, pp. 600–608. https://doi:10.1177/1545968308328726.

"The Rise of Parkinson's Disease." *American Scientist*, https://americanscientist.org/article/the-rise-of-parkinsons-disease. Accessed 4 Oct. 2022.

Schenkman, Margaret, et al. "Effect of High-Intensity Treadmill Exercise on Motor Symptoms in Patients With De Novo Parkinson Disease: A Phase 2 Randomized Clinical Trial." *JAMA Neurology*, vol. 75, no. 2, Feb. 2018, pp. 219–226. https://doi:10.1001/jamaneurol.2017.3517.

Schmidt, Marlene, et al. "Ubiquitin Signalling in Neurodegeneration: Mechanisms and Therapeutic Opportunities." *Cell Death and Differentiation*, vol. 28, no. 2, 28 Feb. 2021, pp. 570–590. https://doi:10.1038/s41418-020-00706-7.

Segura, Carolina, et al. "Effect of a High-Intensity Tandem Bicycle Exercise Program on Clinical Severity, Functional Magnetic Resonance Imaging, and Plasma Biomarkers in Parkinson's Disease." *Frontiers in Neurology*, vol. 11, 24 July 2020, pp. 1–11. https://doi.org/10.3389/fneur.2020.00656. Accessed 9 Aug. 2022.

Silva-Batista, Carla, et al. "Resistance Training with Instability for Patients with Parkinson's Disease." *Medicine and Science in Sports and Exercise*, vol. 48, no. 9, Sept. 2016, pp. 1678–1687. https://doi: 10.1249/MSS.0000000000000945.

Smith, Tyler. "Can Exercise Help Patients Gain Ground on Parkinson's Disease?" *UC Health Today*, 28 Sept. 2021, https://www.uchealth.org/today/can-exercise-help-patients-gain-ground-on-parkinsons-disease/. Accessed 14 Oct. 2022.

Sonne, James W.H., et al. "A Retrospective Analysis of Group-Based Boxing Exercise on Measures of Physical Mobility in Patients with Parkinson Disease." *American Journal of Lifestyle Medicine*, 2021, https://doi:10.1177/15598276211028144.

"SPARX3 Intensifies Efforts Toward a Specific Exercise Prescription in Parkinson's Disease." *Consult QD Blog,* Clevland Clinic, 18 Aug. 2021, https://consultqd.clevelandclinic.org/sparx3-intensifies-efforts-toward-a-specific-exercise-prescription-in-parkinsons-disease/. Accessed 14 Oct. 2022.

"Study in Parkinson's Disease of Exercise Phase 3 Clinical Trial." Northwestern University, 2023, https://www.sparx3pd.com/home. Accessed 3 Oct. 2022.

Suárez-Iglesias, David, et al. "Benefits of Pilates in Parkinson's Disease: A Systematic Review and Meta-Analysis." *Medicina (Kaunas, Lithuania)*, vol. 55, no. 8, 13 Aug. 2019, pp. 1–14. https://doi:10.3390/medicina5508047.

Tajiri, Naoki, et al. "Exercise Exerts Neuroprotective Effects on Parkinson's Disease Model of Rats." *Brain Research*, vol. 1310, 15 Jan. 2010, pp. 200–7. https://doi:10.1016/j.brainres.2009.10.075.

Tanaka, Hirofumi, et al. "Age-Predicted Maximal Heart Rate Revisited." *Journal of the American College of Cardiology*, vol. 37, no. 1, 1 Jan. 2001, pp. 153–6. https://doi.org/10.1016/s0735-1097(00)01054-8.

Thomsen, Birgitte L. C., et al. "Deep Brain Stimulation in Parkinson's Disease: Still Effective After More Than 8 Years." *Movement Disorders Clinical Practice*, vol. 7, no. 7, 21 Sept. 2020, pp. 788–796. https://doi:10.1002/mdc3.13040.

Uc, Ergun Y, et al. "Phase I/II Randomized Trial of Aerobic Exercise in Parkinson Disease in a Community Setting." *Neurology*, vol. 83, no. 5, 29 July 2014, pp. 413–25. https://doi:10.1212/WNL.0000000000000644.

"Unified Parkinson's Disease Rating Scale (UPDRS), Movement Disorders Society (MDS) Modified Unified Parkinson's Disease Rating Scale (MDS-UPDRS)." *American Physical Therapy Association*, 31 Mar. 2018, https://movementdisorders.org/MDS/MDS-Rating-Scales/MDS-Unified-Parkinsons-Disease-Rating-Scale-MDS-UPDRS.htm. Accessed 11 Oct. 2022.

Van der Kolk, Nicolien M., et al. "Effectiveness of Home-Based and Remotely Supervised Aerobic Exercise in Parkinson's Disease: A Double-Blind, Randomized Controlled Trial." *The Lancet. Neurology*, vol. 18, no. 11, 2019, pp. 998–1008. https://doi:10.106/S1474-4422(19)30285-6.

Van Nimwegen, Marlies, et al. "Physical Inactivity in Parkinson's Disease." *Journal of Neurology*, vol. 258, no. 12, Dec. 2011, pp. 2214–21. https://doi:10.1007/s00415-011-6097-7.

Van Puymbroeck, Marieke, et al. "Functional Improvements in Parkinson's Disease Following a Randomized Trial of Yoga." *Evidence-based Complementary and Alternative Medicine, eCAM*, vol. 2018, 2018, pp. 1–8. https://doi:10.1155/2018/8516351.

Vetrano, Davide L, et al. "Sarcopenia in Parkinson Disease: Comparison of Different Criteria and Association with Disease Severity." *Journal of the American Medical Directors Association*, vol. 19, no. 6, June 2018, pp. 523–7. https://doi:10.1016/j.jamda.2017.12.005.

"What is Accreditation?" American Council on Exercise, https://www.acefitness.org/fitness-certifications/accreditation. Accessed 13 Oct. 2022.

Willis, Allison W., et al. "Incidence of Parkinson Disease in North America." *NPJ Parkinson's Disease*, vol. 8, no. 1, 15 Dec. 2022, pp. 1–7. https://doi:10.1038/s41531-022-00410-y.

Yazar, Tamer, et al. "Incidence of Sarcopenia and Dynapenia According to Stage in Patients with Idiopathic Parkinson's Disease." *Neurological Sciences*, vol. 39, no. 8, 12 May 2018, pp.1415–1421. https://doi:10.1007/s10072-018-3439-6.

Zhang, Xiaoqun, and Karima Chergui. "Dopamine Depletion of the Striatum Causes a Cell-Type Specific Reorganization of GluN2B-and GluN2D-Containing NMDA Receptors." *Neuropharmacology*, vol. 92, May 2015, pp. 108–115. https:// doi:10.1016/j.neuropharm.2015.01.007.

Made in the USA
Middletown, DE
22 August 2024

59576915R00124